Making Sense of Life

Jason and Patsy Taylor
Ph. 630-557-0097
46 W611 Main St. Rd.
P. O. Box 128
Kaneville, Il 60144

Other books in this series

Making Sense of Life

When Our Real Home Is Heaven

John Guest

Foreword by Steve Brown

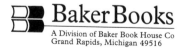

Baker Books

A Division of Baker Book House Co
Grand Rapids, Michigan 49516

© 1994 by John Guest
The first edition of this book appeared in 1988 under the title *This World Is Not My Home.*

Published by Baker Books
a division of Baker Book House Company
P.O. Box 6287, Grand Rapids, MI 49516-6287

ISBN 0-8010-3867-7

Printed in the United States of America

Unless otherwise indicated, all Scripture in this volume is from the Revised Standard Version of the Bible, copyright 1946, 1952, 1971, and 1973 by the Division of Christian Education of the National Council of the Churches of Christ in the United States of America. Other versions used include the King James Version (KJV), The New Testament in the Language of Today (Beck), and the New International Version (NIV).

I will be forever grateful to
Tom and Alice Frearson, who first introduced
me to the United States of America. They inspired
me to stay and over the years they have similarly
inspired my ministry. Subsequently,
I owe my American
citizenship and my dear wife, Kathie, and
our family to their influence.

Contents

Foreword

The English philosopher Thomas Hobbes described the life of man as "solitary, poor, nasty, brutish, and short." There was a time when my philosophy, boiled down to its essence, was pretty much summed up in that statement. I had read and become enamored with Aibert Camus (French philosopher, novelist, and dramatist), who suggested that the only question with which a thinking human being should deal was the question of whether or not one should commit suicide. He said that there was no ultimate meaning to life and, if one wanted meaning, one had to create that meaning for oneself.

If your meaning consisted in sexual gratification, building hospitals, or feeding hungry people, it really didn't matter because it had no ultimate significance. It was your meaning and when you died, your meaning would die too.

That was a very painful and difficult time of my life. I didn't know it, but the "hound of heaven" was beginning his stalking of my soul. He had begun by leading me to ask the right questions: Who am I? What is life all about? Where am I going? Does any of this make sense? Does any of this matter? Once the questions were asked, he provided the answers. Not only that, he *became* the answers.

If you have begun your quest, I have some exciting news for you: What God begins, he always completes, and the fact of its beginning is a promise of its completion. In other words, you have embarked on a journey of meaning, joy, and discovery, and the fact that you have begun it is a promise from God that he will complete it. *Making Sense of Life* will be a good guide for you and your journey into the light. John Guest has been there; he has asked the same questions you have asked; he has known the pain of thinking that maybe all that is, is an accident. And, having made the journey himself, with great compassion, honesty, and joy, he will be your guide as you make it.

This isn't just a book that answers questions for those who search. It is also a book for those of us who have found the answers but have sometimes forgotten. I'm told that whenever a sports team begins to falter, coaches tell athletes that they must go back to the basics. That is a good idea for Christians too.

We are too busy. Sometimes the "busyness" covers the fact that we don't hear the "soft sound of sandaled feet" anymore. Sometimes the "stuff" we have acquired and the busy (even religious) lives that we lead blind us to the One who loved us, who forgave us, who brought us together, who sent us into the world, and who promised to get us home "before the dark."

When the harsh bark of the con men, the false faces of the actors, the glitter of the trinkets, the clack of the word processors, and the glare of the neon signs are more real than God, Christians—even "mature" Christians—need to get quiet and remember what this thing is all about.

This is a book of remembering what the One who has called us would tell his own about the meaning of life. It is a book Christians ought to go back to often so we don't forget that the "family secrets" are simple, profound, and filled with the laughter of God for a sour world.

I commend it to you.

Steve Brown

Introduction

've chosen to build this book loosely around the frame of Paul's epistle to the Christians at Philippi. Of all Paul's letters to churches, this is his most personal and his most joyful. In contrast to Paul's letters to others, in which he berates or chastises readers at length, this piece of correspondence offers one point of encouragement after another.

He's writing old and particularly generous friends; he wishes he could be with them, speaking face to face instead of writing words to be delivered by a mutual friend. But for the time being that's impossible, as he's not a free man. He's in Rome, it seems, under house arrest and awaiting trial.

Because this letter is so personal, it rambles from one issue to another and back around again. (Isn't that always the case when you write good friends?) And because his missive jumps from this to that, my discussion of some of Paul's concerns follows an outline that is mine, not his. But right here, I'd like to start where Paul starts. He addresses this letter to "all the saints in Christ Jesus who are at Philippi" (1:1).

These saints to whom he wrote were not some lofty heroes who were, as the saying goes, so heavenly minded they were no earthly good. They were ordinary people who lived in an ordinary world full of challenges and obstacles not much different from those we face today.

If Paul were alive now this letter addressed to the Philippians could well be his message to my own church. Or it might be meant for a church in your community—one to which you belong or one that would welcome you should you look to them for fellowship. The saints were simply Christians—people who were in Christ.

As Paul wrote his letter to the saints, so I address this book to you saints who have entrusted your lives to Jesus Christ.

But I go one step beyond that and invite all sinners as well to read these pages. For you I pray that God might open his floodgates of mercy and, more, that you will be ready to receive the grace he offers as a free gift.

1

Citizen of a New Land

I t was a pleasant fall day in September 1974. In many ways the day was like any other since I'd moved to Pittsburgh six years earlier. I got up, shaved, ate my Wheaties, looked at the newspaper headlines and briefly reviewed my day's schedule with my wife, Kathie. But in one major way this day was like none other I'd ever lived.

Late that morning, I drove down into the heart of the city, to the massive, marble federal courthouse on Grant Street. As I parked the car and hurried toward the appointed room number, I became increasingly aware of other people—by themselves and with families—heading in the same direction as I. We were as different as people can be: Our appearances and our accents betrayed our origins.

As a white, Anglo-Saxon Protestant with a clear British accent, I was in the minority. Many people gathering in the large hall were East Asians, speaking to one another with chopped sing-song words. Some quiet Indian women had red dots painted on their foreheads. A few Latino men gestured with their hands as they spoke what I recognized as Spanish. I don't know how many countries were represented that day, but where we were from was of no consequence when compared to what we were about to become: new citizens of the United States of America.

I was born in England and lived near London all through my childhood, moving to the United States when I was thirty. In time, of my own free will, I chose to give up my English citizenship and commit myself to this great nation, which said, "Yes, we will have you as one of our sons if you commit yourself to our flag and to the republic for which it stands."

So on that bright September day, before a roomful of witnesses, I raised my right hand, disavowed my allegiance to the land of my birth, and swore my allegiance to the United States of America. I was ecstatic. I had a new home. I was a new person in that I had walked into that courthouse an Englishman and walked out an American.

Now let me tell you about another day in my life. I was younger then—eighteen. The sun dawns over the London horizon hours before it gets to Pittsburgh, so you might say that my days of youth started earlier than they do now. A few other details of my morning routine have changed as I've grown older, but suffice it to say that this spring day was rather typical until evening, when a classmate and I went to London's Harringay Arena to hear a young American evangelist, Billy Graham, preach.

A couple of years before, a coworker had tried to tell me that Jesus had died to give me a new life, but the words hadn't sunk in. More recently, when I'd started going to church in order to win the heart of a girl I wanted to impress, I'd heard the same thing from the minister in my neighborhood. And now this Bible-holding, finger-pointing preacher was saying it again: Jesus loved me. Graham wanted me to turn my back on my old life and start new. As he was winding down he asked people who wanted to accept Christ to get up out of their seats and make a public statement of their decision by walking to the front of the arena.

I remember being horrified at the boldness of the American-style altar call and equally amazed at the crowd that gathered across the front of the hall. At my seat I stood tight through the first verse of "Just As I Am." Although I knew that I should put my life in God's hands, my pride glued my feet to the floor—that is, until the second verse. Then, just as I was, I stepped into the aisle and walked toward the praying evangelist, though he was not really my destination. No, I was walking toward Jesus, giving him my fragmented past, my hopeful future, my loyalty and allegiance.

That night I placed myself in Jesus' hands. I prayed, asking God to forgive my sins and accept me into his fold. I left that arena ecstatic. I actually danced down the streets of London, whirling myself around the lampposts—the kind of scene you think happens only in the movies. At the very core of my being I was a new person. I had walked into that service a child of Adam and Eve; I walked out a child of God.

When describing this type of transformation to Nicodemus, Jesus used the phrase that has become trivialized in recent years—"born again." He said, "Truly, truly, I say to you, unless one is born anew, he cannot see the kingdom of God" (John 3:3).

When describing the transformation to a woman of Samaria who was drawing water from a well, Jesus used a different metaphor. He said, "Every one who drinks of this water will thirst again, but whoever drinks of the water that I shall give him will never thirst; the water that I shall give him will become in him a spring of water welling up to eternal life" (John 4:13–14).

In his letter written to Christians in the city of Philippi, the apostle Paul painted yet another word picture of the Christian life. "Our commonwealth is in heaven," he said (Phil. 3:20). Other translations give a more clear and accurate rendition of the Greek. The New English Bible reads, "We . . . are citizens of heaven," and the New American Standard Bible says, "Our citizenship is in heaven."

On that warm May night when I was eighteen, my citizenship changed from one kingdom to another, just as surely as it did twenty years later when I stood in front of a United States federal judge. I turned my back on the kingdom into which I was born—this world and its temporarily powerful ruler, Satan—and pledged my allegiance to the kingdom of heaven, ruled by Jesus the Messiah.

Jesus the King

The New Testament is full of references to Jesus as king, but two are especially significant. That royal title was given to him at the time of his birth and at the time of his death.

When the angel Gabriel told Mary that she would have a son fathered by the Spirit of God, Gabriel said that "the Lord God will give to him the throne of his father David, and he will reign over the house of Jacob for ever; and of his kingdom there will be no end" (Luke 1:32–33).

I'm not sure Mary had any idea what those words meant until more than thirty years later, after Pilate, the Roman governor of Judea, directly asked Jesus if the treason charges against him were true. At Jesus' trial, Pilate asked, "Are you the King of the Jews?" And what did Jesus answer? "My kingship is not of this world; if my kingship were of this world, my servants would fight, that I might not be handed over to the Jews; but my kingship is not from the world." Pilate wanted a straighter answer and kept pushing the question: "So you are a king?" (John 18:33–37).

As the Jerusalem Bible translates it, Jesus answered, "Yes, I am a king. I was born for this, I came into the world for this: to bear witness to the truth; and all who are on the side of truth listen to my voice" (v. 37).

Within hours of that conversation Jesus was torturously dying as if he were a traitor. He was nailed to a tree trunk underneath a sign written by Pilate himself: "Jesus of Nazareth, the King of the Jews."

Of course, if Jesus had been a king of an earthly state (or of no state at all), the story would have ended that afternoon when he was pronounced dead at the scene. At the time there seemed to be no question about his demise, as the soldiers treated him differently from the men on either side of him who were also crucified. As sundown approached, soldiers broke the legs of the two other convicts; they wanted to hasten the hour of death so families could bury the dead before the Sabbath brought the city to a standstill. But with Jesus, they took another tack. With a spear they pierced his side, evidently to ensure that the dead was dead.

On that Friday afternoon, Jesus was wrapped in grave clothes and laid in a tomb sealed with a huge boulder. The place was guarded round the clock by several Roman soldiers.

But, as I said, the story didn't end on Friday. What happened the next Sunday morning proved Jesus' lordship over a kingdom that is above and beyond this physical and fallen world.

The Miracle of Miracles

Early on that Sunday morning, which we now call Easter, several devoted, grieving women went to Jesus' tomb to continue the burial ritual; they carried aromatic spices with which they would anoint the decaying body. But much to their surprise they didn't find a cold corpse. They discovered empty grave clothes and a walking, talking, breathing Jesus.

He addressed them by name. He showed them the nail holes in his palms. He sent them back into town to tell the other disciples what they'd seen—that he was alive. He who had been dead for three days rose from the grave.

There have always been scoffers, people who have claimed that Jesus did not rise from the dead. Some have claimed that the body was stolen by the disciples. This theory seems to have been planted and spread immediately by the Jewish priests in Jerusalem. Matthew 28 claims that the chief priests paid off the Roman guards who reported the resurrection to them. The guards were told to "tell people, 'His disciples came by night and stole him away while we were asleep.'" Matthew continues, "So they took the money and did as they were directed; and this story has been spread among the Jews to this day" (Matt. 28:13, 15).

But think about it for a minute. Neither the Romans nor the Jews—nor the disciples, for that matter—claimed to have turned up the body. Quite the contrary. Within a few months of the resurrection, the screws tightened around the disciples because they wouldn't stop preaching that Jesus had risen.

James the brother of John was the first of the disciples to be martyred for his stand, and over the years all but John were violently killed for their bold witness—while John died in exile on an isolated island where he wouldn't cause anybody any trouble. Despite imprisonment, beatings, and death threats, the apostles didn't lead anyone to a decomposed body. They just kept preaching that Jesus was alive and had conquered death.

They spoke with conviction that was based on their own eye witness. In the forty days between his resurrection and his ascension into heaven, Jesus had repeatedly visited them. He'd eaten with them; he'd invited them to touch his open wounds. He'd explained to them some of his stories that had previously seemed pointless or beyond their grasp. They'd then watched as he physically left the earth, ascending into the heavens before their very eyes.

Those apostles knew where their Lord was. They knew he was not lying in a cave or buried under a mound of dirt. Otherwise, they would have memorialized the place where he lay. Graveyards and death sites have always been made into monuments of the giants who have fallen. This was true even in early history; the pyramids are the most obvious of such ancient shrines. In fact, guarding against this human tendency seems to be the reason why God saw that old Moses died alone. Deuteronomy 34:6 says that God himself buried Moses in Moab, and "no man knows the place of his burial to this day."

Our own culture is amazingly obsessed with such memorial sites. An eternal flame, for example, marks the grave of John Kennedy. But presidents aren't the only heroes with memorials.

I remember being fascinated with James Dean. That dates me, of course. Some of you don't even know who he was. He starred in some wonderful movies, such as "East of Eden" and "Rebel Without a Cause." When you walked out of one of his movies you went home broody, moody, and intense, somehow walking in the spirit of the man. But then in 1955 he was killed in an automobile accident in California, and for years after his death a group of fans would gather at the site of the crash and have a memorial service. Look at Elvis Presley—his grave has become a tourist attraction.

Now the same thing, of course, eventually happened with Jesus' tomb—it became a shrine and a place of pilgrimage—but not in the lifetime of Jesus' apostles. They did not have a morbid fixation on the death of Jesus; rather, their lives were consumed with the reality of—and driven by the power of—the resurrected Jesus.

So much for the dead body theory, but what about the swoon theory? Some people like to claim that Jesus never really died, and thus his return to the land of the living was a natural rather than a supernatural phenomenon. But this makes even less sense than the story cooked up by the Jerusalem priests.

Do you think those original followers of Jesus would have been inspired to rally around a whipped, gasping man who woke from a three-day, stone-cold swoon looking like death warmed over? They would have had to nurse him back to health and they would have *known* that he was a loser—like every other loser who had claimed to be their king. The scenario could never have inspired a movement that has changed—and is still changing—the world. They would have carted him off to the hills of Galilee and returned to their fishing nets.

A tidbit about Jesus' own family fits in here. Acts 15 records what is considered to be the first major council of the young but growing church. Christians from the various parts of the then-evangelized world gathered for a meeting, and the obvious chairman of the convocation was James the brother of Jesus.

More often than not, a person's immediate family is the most skeptical about a conversion or a miraculous event. During Jesus' lifetime, his family seemed to have questions about his message and lifestyle. Tradition claims that James the brother of Jesus didn't become a disciple until *after* the resurrection, and that claim in itself carries considerable weight. When a family member is convinced, having first been a skeptic, you know you are dealing with authentic evidence.

Yet a third theory says that the disciples, overcome with their grief, suffered hallucinations and convinced themselves that their leader had returned from the dead. That line of thought might hold some water if Jesus had been seen alive by only one person at a time—that is, if no one else in the room could verify what an individual had witnessed. But you can't get six or twenty or five hundred, as recorded in 1 Corinthians 15, to risk their lives claiming they've seen the same hallucination. And in any case, no psychiatrist will ever give credence to the possibility of "mass hallucinations."

Ultimately, the theories not based on fact fall by the wayside, and the truth remains: Jesus rose from the dead, and in doing so he proved the extent and power of his rule. He was born, he died, and he came back to life as a king who reigns over life—and death—itself.

Jesus is the only king who offers life—citizenship in a kingdom that never will be defeated, that never will end— to anyone who desires to become a subject. And he makes that offer to us—just as we are. No courses required. No physical or AIDS blood test required. No nationality quotas. No security clearance.

A Skeptic Is Convinced

That's made clear in the New Testament telling of an amazing conversion story. The conversion of Saul of Tarsus might be comparable to a news story reporting that the Ayatollah Khomeini had become a Christian. In addition, Saul (later called Paul) started preaching on a grand scale, as if the Ayatollah were to start conducting Billy Graham-style evangelistic crusades, calling people to give their lives to Christ!

In the days right after Jesus' resurrection, Paul had been a militant leader of the organized Jewish traditionalists who were ready to kill followers of Christ in order to hold on to the pure and traditional religion. Acts 8:3 and 9:1 and 2 are rather condemning: "Saul laid waste the church, and entering house after house, he dragged off men and women and committed them to prison. . . . But Saul, still breathing threats and murders against the disciples of the Lord, went to the high priest and asked him for letters to the synagogues at Damascus, so that if he found any belonging to the Way, men or women, he might bring them bound to Jerusalem."

On that trip to Damascus to "lay waste" the church there, Saul was suddenly struck blind with a flash of light and awakened with a flash of truth. In that moment he saw Jesus, who spoke directly to him: "Saul, Saul, why do you persecute me?" Then Jesus clearly identified himself. "I am

Jesus," he said, "whom you are persecuting" (Acts 9:4–5). Paul suddenly had reason to believe that Jesus had risen from the dead. From that day on, his witness for Christ was as bold as that of the original apostles who'd repeatedly seen Jesus in the days between his resurrection and his ascension.

As you can imagine, the disciples were a little skeptical at first, thinking a faked conversion would be the perfect trick for Saul to play—to draw them out of hiding so he could drag them off to prison. But through a vision the Lord told one Christian leader in Damascus, Ananias, that Paul was a changed man. And besides that, the disciples watched him; Acts 9:22 states that "Saul increased all the more in strength, and confounded the Jews who lived in Damascus by proving that Jesus was the Christ"—that is, the long-awaited Messiah and king.

In the next verse it was the Jews who were plotting to kill Saul. So he had to escape in the dead of night by hiding in a basket and being lowered by Christians over the city wall. The hunter had become the hunted.

The transformation of Saul was radical, even revolutionary, for he was the greatest missionary the Christian church has ever known. He traveled into Europe to spread the gospel and, even more than that, he wrote most of what became our New Testament.

But any change that came in Saul, or Paul, came as he laid his sin at the foot of Jesus' cross—no previous requirements necessary. As Paul did that, he felt the power of the resurrection of Jesus, to which he referred years later when he wrote to the Philippian church (Phil. 3:10). The power of the resurrection is not something that only raises dead bodies from the grave. It is the same power that can transform lives and circumstances.

The Power Is Ours

That's the way God still works. I'll never forget the conversion story a Jewish Christian man once told me. He was at the end of his rope. He'd lost his business in Miami and was flying to New York City for a job interview, though he had little hope of being hired.

As he walked through the New York airport he was contemplating suicide. Suddenly he was surprised when a stranger walked up to him and slipped a card into his hand. It read, "You look as if you need help. Give me a call."

That evening when he got to his hotel room, he started looking at the Gideon Bible lying open on the nightstand. One thing led to another and he dialed the number on the card. As you might suspect, the stranger told him about Jesus, the Messiah.

The unemployed man listened and thought this over for quite some time, until he became intellectually convinced that Jesus had risen from the dead, that he was the Messiah. But it was not until he was back in Florida that the full weight of that truth struck him in a way reminiscent of Saul's conversion experience. As he was thinking heavily on his newfound Messiah the car he was driving was suddenly filled with a bright light. He told me, "I was so overwhelmed by the presence of Jesus in my car that I had to pull over and just sit there."

Overwhelming a sinner with a bright light is not the Lord's usual mode of operation. That's not what happened to me or to most Christians I know or hear about. The tug of the Holy Spirit is usually internal and much like a kindly father beckoning you to come home. It is like the Statue of Liberty, lifting high a welcoming torch of freedom. Just as the statue beckons, "Give me your tired, your poor," Jesus says, "Come to me, all who labor and are heavy laden, and I will give you rest" (Matt. 11:28).

Pledging Our Allegiance

The citizenship God offers us is ours for the taking. It is a free gift. We simply have to believe that Jesus' death and resurrection are the doorway from death to life. It means we have to believe that Jesus, God in human form, took our sins on himself and gave us his righteousness (2 Cor. 5:21). It means we have to pledge new loyalties to God himself— to his love, his truth, his goodness, his righteousness.

I've heard the story of a man who lived in America during the Civil War. Having sympathy with both the Northern and Southern causes, he never really chose sides. In fact, he wore a blue blazer and gray trousers as a sign of his state of mind. But, as you can imagine, neither army owned him as its own, and ultimately the man was shot at by both Union and Confederate troops.

Back in the 1960s a slogan was frequently bantered around: "Not to decide is to decide." The truth of that statement couldn't be applied more aptly than to citizenship. Until I chose to be an American citizen—and America chose to accept me—I was a citizen of England, the land of my parentage and my birth. I would have died as a subject of England had I not decided to change my status and my loyalties. In the same way, I would have died a citizen of this world that is temporarily under the thumb of Satan, had I not made a decision—at a Billy Graham crusade in 1954.

In Sunday school many youngsters learn a pledge of allegiance to the Christian flag: "I pledge allegiance to the Christian flag and to the Savior for whose kingdom it stands. One Savior, crucified, risen, and coming again, with life and liberty for all who believe."

Right now, whether you're lounging in your home, riding a crosstown bus or waiting for a dentist to pull a tooth, you can become a citizen of heaven. The decision doesn't call for a change of residence; it doesn't mean that the king will immediately summon you to his other-worldly capital city.

It means this world is no longer "home" to you. As the old gospel song says, "This world is not my home, I'm just a-passing through . . . I can't feel at home in this world anymore." Why? Because our eyes are on and our concerns are with Jesus, the sovereign ruler whose kingdom is not of this world.

When writing to the Corinthian church, Paul said, "Behold, now is the acceptable time; behold, now is the day of salvation" (2 Cor. 6:2). He's ready to receive you. Are you ready to decide?

A Prayer

Jesus, thank you for opening your arms to me, for becoming human and taking my sins on your perfect self so that the door to citizenship is open to me. Right now I want to make a decision—to turn my back on my sin and to pledge my allegiance to you and your kingdom. Help me as I begin my new journey to live a life that is worthy of my citizenship in heaven. Amen.

2

A Privileged People

If I had been God, I might have ordered the world differently. I think I would have provided my people with a tamper-free world, a utopia where life was serene and predictable (though never boring) and perfect.

Well, that seems to be what God has in mind for his people—eventually. But here you and I sit, somewhere in the long and short (depending on your outlook) "in the meantime" that we call life.

Right before his death, Jesus prayed for his disciples using phrases that seem contradictory yet make sense when they're understood in terms of being citizens of heaven while we remain here on earth. In John 17:16 Jesus says of his disciples, "They are not of the world, even as I am not of the world." And in the previous verse he says, "I do not pray that thou shouldst take them out of the world, but that thou shouldst keep them from the evil one." His disciples were not of this world, yet they were to remain for a time in this world to live as citizens loyal to their heavenly king.

The first words in Arthur Simon's book *Christian Faith and Public Policy: No Grounds for Divorce* say it all— "Christians have dual citizenship. We are citizens of God's kingdom and citizens of an earthly country." Being "in the world" is the reality we live with temporarily. And as long as we're here in what is a foreign land to us—as long as history has not yet come to the point when Satan has been bound and the earth has been made new—our heavenly citizenship, like our physical citizenship, comes with both privileges and responsibilities.

Before we look at some of the privileges we Christians enjoy, let's consider what the privilege of citizenship meant to the apostle Paul and his Philippian friends.

A Roman Colony

When we think of Bible lands in New Testament times we often think of a repressive, ugly occupation by the Romans. The army of Rome had swept down and captured Galilee and Judea. There was no question about who was in charge—and who wasn't. The relatively few Romans in Palestine had power and preferred privilege that came from their connection to the mother country. The native Jewish population was treated with contempt and as subjects—not as citizens.

But things were a little different in Philippi, a city in Macedonia, a region that has long since been divided up into what is now Bulgaria, Yugoslavia, and Greece. While Galilee and Judea were occupied and "out back" Roman territories, Philippi was a colony, more valued and prestigious.

Rome established these colonies at major crossroads. They had the appearance and the flavor of Roman cities. Many of the residents were military veterans and their families, sent to the colonies in reward for their career service. On the soldiers' retirement, these families were also awarded Roman citizenship, the ultimate privilege that assured them of physical and judicial security. They were safe from outside marauders. If accused of crime, they could appeal to a system that guaranteed due process of law.

Because of Philippi's privileged status, the Christians who lived there had a unique and personal understanding of what citizenship was all about. In the introduction to his

Daily Study Bible on Philippians, William Barclay goes so far as to say that Philippians 3:20, "We . . . are citizens of heaven" (NEB), really means that we are "a colony of heaven." Barclay continues, "Nowhere were men prouder of being Roman citizens than in these colonies. And such was Philippi."

Paul Appeals

Paul himself, though not from Philippi, was a privileged Roman citizen. At least twice he appealed to his rights as granted by law. One of these times he was in Philippi, on a preaching mission with a coworker named Silas.

One afternoon on their way to a prayer meeting, Paul and Silas were harassed by a fortune-telling slave girl who was demon-possessed. This went on for several days, and when Paul had had just about enough, he turned to the girl and commanded the evil spirit to leave her in Jesus' name. This release delighted the girl but infuriated her owners, who'd lost their "hope of gain," as Luke says in Acts 16:19.

Now Paul's Jewishness was obvious to these men, but his Roman citizenship was not. He seemed to be an unprotected foreigner, so they took him to the town square, called out the justice of the peace and said, "These men are Jews and they are disturbing our city. They advocate customs which it is not lawful for us Romans to accept or practice" (Acts 16:20–21).

Those accusations were serious enough that the police were called in and given orders to beat Paul and Silas heartily with rods, throw them in prison and lock their feet in stocks. But hours later, about midnight, as Paul and Silas were singing hymns and praying, an "act of God" changed the course of the story. An earthquake shook the prison, forcing all the stock and door locks. A prisonful of convicts was loose, and just the thought of his probable fate made the jailer despair. He'd raised his sword and was about to pierce his own chest when Paul called out to him and assured him that no one had run away.

Paul's testimony on that one night—his joy and his integrity—prompted the Roman jailer to ask a pointed question: "What must I do to be saved?" (v. 30). Paul and Silas's answer was just as straight: "Believe in the Lord Jesus" (v. 31). Before dawn the missionaries had baptized the jailer's whole family; as new citizens of heaven, the converts wanted to give this visible witness to their change of loyalty.

It's likely that this jailer became one of the leaders in the Philippian church to which Paul addressed his later letter. But our story here really is about Paul, who's been charged with anti-Roman activities.

When the justice of the peace found out that Paul and Silas had maintained order in the prison during the earthquake, he quietly ordered that the charges be dropped. But Paul resisted that plan. To the jailer he said, "They have beaten us publicly, uncondemned, men who are Roman citizens, and have thrown us into prison; and do they now cast us out secretly? No! let them come themselves and take us out." Luke, the historian, continues, "The police reported these words to the magistrates, and they were afraid when they heard that they were *Roman* citizens; so they came and apologized to them. And they took them out and asked them to leave the city" (vv. 37–39, italics added). Which is exactly what Paul and Silas did.

Much later, when Paul was arrested in Jerusalem, he again appealed to the privileges of citizenship. As he was about to be "examined by scourging, to find out why they shouted thus against him," Paul asked the nearest guard, "Is it lawful for you to scourge a man who is a Roman citizen, and uncondemned?" Those words seemed to work like magic. The soldier went to the tribune, who spoke to Paul himself. When the official said, with some pride, "I bought this citizenship for a large sum," Paul did him one better with a quick "I was born a citizen" (Acts 22:24–28).

Again, Luke says that the Roman officials were afraid for themselves for having ill-treated *a citizen.* The very next day a city-wide Jewish council was called to examine the charges against Paul, and eventually Paul traveled across the Mediterranean to Rome itself to appeal his case to Caesar.

Our Own Privileges

It's obvious that citizenship did—and still does—include privilege. The United States is probably on better terms with Canada than with any other country. But let a U.S. citizen just try to drive across the border and apply for work in Toronto. Immediately that person will realize the employment opportunity benefits that come with being one of "our own," or of "their own," as the case may be.

This same principle applies to citizens of the kingdom of heaven. If I were to discuss in depth all the privileges that are ours through Christ, the size of this book would scare readers away. But let's look at a few rights that are unequivocally ours when we become Christians.

We Know Who We Are and Where We're Going

Let me tell you a little about my childhood. In one word, we were poor, shamefully poor. My father died when I was seven, during World War II. At first I'd walk along the streets, looking into every man's face, trying to find my dad. I couldn't believe he was dead.

The British government was busy fighting Germany and couldn't spend a great deal of effort or money on the welfare of its own people. Mother had three sons to feed. I remember being thrilled when a neighbor brought over a lowly head of cabbage and when we received secondhand clothes from the States. I got ahold of a pair of knickerbockers and made my mother cut them off so I could wear them as if they were trousers. They looked ridiculous—they were too big for me—but I was glad to have them.

At one point I remember wearing a pair of girls' shoes to school. It was either that or no shoes at all. I did take a little piece of glass decoration off the top of them so they wouldn't look so feminine. Another time I remember not being able to play soccer on the school team because I didn't have soccer boots.

Kids of every generation are downright mean in their judgments of who's cool and who's not. I may have been cold, but I wasn't cool. The stares and the titters of my classmates and my heart's ache to be on the school soccer team, convinced me that I was made of inferior stuff.

As a result, I spent my youth trying to prove to the world and to myself that I was somebody—somebody who didn't need to take a back seat to anybody else. It's the old "anything you can do, I can do better" syndrome that flows from a sense of inferiority.

Nevertheless, that's a part of my youth that I've shed, like a snake sheds a skin, and without the help of a psychotherapist. It happened the night I asked the Lord Jesus to come into my life. That night I knew I was a person of great worth and dignity. I was no longer a fatherless child—or a fatherless grown man.

No, I was the son, the heir, of a king. I was a privileged citizen. Look at what Paul says in Romans 8: "For all who are led by the Spirit of God are sons of God. For you did not receive the spirit of slavery to fall back into fear, but you have received the spirit of sonship. When we cry, 'Abba! Father!' it is the Spirit himself bearing witness with our spirit that we are children of God, and if children, then heirs, heirs of God and fellow heirs with Christ, provided we suffer with him in order that we may also be glorified with him" (vv. 14–17).

If I was a child of God, if I was a fellow heir with Christ, then I had a dignity that was legitimate. I had a dignity that came from outside myself but that was planted within me. It was not—like possessions or positions—something that was subject to change without notice. It was not based on shifting moods, like the admiration of friends or even family. It was founded on God, a rock that would be solid and sure—through any earthquake or any atomic bomb blast. My new identity and dignity were not my own but that of God in me.

When I was fifteen I would have laughed if someone had told me that I'd eventually be a spiritual leader in one of the wealthiest communities in the world. But just as absurd would have been the notion that I would move among my parishioners and among the city leaders without feeling inferior to them. My sense of worth is nothing short of a miracle of God's grace—which he wants every citizen of his kingdom to realize and enjoy.

That sense of worth was also tied to my sense of destiny. Think about it: If there is no destination, there is no destiny. I see life as a big, beautiful picture. I like to think of this grand design as a large mural—a tremendous landscape that includes leaping animals, working and picnicking people, maybe a country scene in the foreground and a city in the distance. When you stand back from a long mural and look at it start to finish, you see the flow of it. You see the artistic genius at work. But if you walk up and put your nose to it and focus on one square foot of the total picture, you have no idea what that little piece is all about. If the canvas is gray and black at that point, you tend to despair.

To put it in a neat and tidy phrase, the context gives meaning to the content. It's true of a mural and it's true of life. But sadly enough, many people look at one small piece of their lives and conclude that life is meaningless. They ask, "Is that all there is?"

Before I was a Christian, when I was a young teen, I had it all worked out. I didn't know the terms *existentialist* or *relativist*, but I had it figured out: When they bury you, I thought, it's all over. I remember thinking, No wonder most adults appear to be so miserable. They've done all there is to do. They have all the sex they want. They have their jobs, their homes, their gardens. They can go fishing and relax when they want.

I looked into my future and picked what I considered a grown-up age: twenty-five. By the time I'm twenty-five, I thought, I'll have done it all. I'll be bored and miserable, just like all the adults up and down my street.

That kind of thinking is one of the things that drove me to Christ. Paul understood that frame of mind when he said, "If for this life only we have hoped in Christ, we are of all men most to be pitied. But in fact Christ has been raised from the dead" (1 Cor. 15:19–20). Because he lives, life makes sense; I have a reason to get out of bed in the morning—even though I've lived more than double those imagined twenty-five years. Because he lives, I know that good has already defeated evil. Because he lives, I know that this world is not my home. There's a grand and eternal mural that is more beautiful than anything I can imagine—and I have a significant place in that picture.

Courage

This new sense of identity, dignity, and destiny that comes with citizenship is closely connected to another privilege: courage. Sir Winston Churchill gave the world a statement that's nearly good enough to be in the Bible: "Without courage all other virtues lose their meaning." In other words, what is truth if you don't have the courage to speak it? What is righteousness if you don't have the courage to live it? What is love if you don't have the courage to make yourself vulnerable? Without courage the other virtues lose their meaning, their worth, and their power.

Courage is a theme that runs throughout the whole Bible. When God is talking to his people he says repeatedly, "Don't be afraid. I am God, and I am with you." Since Jesus' resurrection and the coming of the Holy Spirit, that message to us is spoken even more emphatically: "Don't be afraid. I am God, and I am in you."

Do you remember the words from Romans 8 about our being children and heirs? Verse 15 said, "For you did not receive the spirit of slavery to fall back into fear." In 2 Timothy 1:7 Paul says something similar: "God did not give us a spirit of timidity" or fear. Fear is not a part of our inheritance.

Psalm 27:14 included a great admonition: "Let your heart take courage." Frankly, it takes courage for a heart to let go of the past—the feelings of worthlessness and of guilt— and to accept God's grace.

Have you ever watched a trapeze act in the circus? It's not just a matter of sitting or standing or even hanging by the knees from a swing suspended high above the ground. That seems challenging enough, but the real act is when the trapeze artists fly from one swing to another.

Over on the left a man might be swinging back and forth, dangling by his knees. On the right, a woman does the same. Suddenly she lets go and flies toward his outstretched hands. I can't say that I've ever tried this feat, but I can tell you that letting go of one's own trapeze and falling into thin air, trusting that your partner will grab you, calls for a spurt of courage.

We can find a parallel to this feat in our spiritual lives. Most of us would rather not let go of our high-flying swing and trust ourselves to Jesus. Too scary, we say, to "let go and let God" grab hold of us so he can make a spectacular production of our lives.

I know Christians whose lives revolve around the negative feelings they hold on to. They are so down on themselves that guilt and depression and that "I'm not good enough" feeling are their roommates. They wouldn't know what to do with themselves if they weren't feeling self-condemnation, which, according to Paul, is not what God has in mind for his children. Romans 8:1 says, "There is therefore now no condemnation for those who are in Christ Jesus."

Dwight L. Moody, the great American evangelist of the nineteenth century, told a wonderful story of his young daughter coming to him and asking his forgiveness for something she'd done wrong. Her father immediately said, "Yes, darling, of course you are forgiven." Now he thought this matter was over, but the next day the girl was back at his side, again asking forgiveness for the same offense. A second time he answered, "Yes, of course you are forgiven. I told you that yesterday." But she came back the third day, and even a fourth day, expressing the same concern, "Daddy, will you forgive me for what I did last week?" By this time the father wasn't pleased with what he sensed in his daughter. Why, he wondered, doesn't she believe that I forgave her when she first asked? Why does she keep coming back, so full of remorse? Doesn't she believe me?

This story raises the same question for me as it did for Moody: Is this how we respond to God's forgiveness of our sins? The new life Christ gives us requires that we reach out in courage and accept God's favor, the grace, even life, that he offers.

Proclaiming the Gospel

For the sake of an ordered table of contents, I've chosen to look at some of the privileges of our citizenship, then move on to our responsibilities. But I'll be the first to point out a flaw in my outline: On close examination, the two categories often overlap. Consider courage, for example. Is it a privilege or a responsibility? I've chosen to say it's a privilege; yet I well know that sometimes "Be not afraid" is a hard command I am responsible to obey by faith—for often I'm scared stiff!

Sharing the gospel of Jesus Christ is yet another privilege of those who are citizens of heaven. Nevertheless, proclaiming the good news—which is what the word *gospel* means—is like courage in that it's also a responsibility. For myself, I can't name any activity that gives more joy and honor than the satisfaction of knowing that someone has been introduced to the Lord, and that's really what sharing the gospel is all about. But there are times when I'm terrified by the task.

Back in the bad old days of the late sixties and early seventies, I was traveling with a rock group trying to evangelize university students. I was at Kent State about three weeks before the uprising there in which several students were killed.

Now this was evangelism with a vengeance. You could hear our amplified music four or five city blocks away. We were gathering great crowds and telling them how Jesus had turned our lives around. We wanted to impress a radical message on the minds of these students who were driven by the radical politics of that generation.

After one performance, a chap from SDS (Students for a Democratic Society—a radical leftist student organization) stepped out of the crowd, came up to me and said, "Hey, man, where are you at?" I can still see him, bandanna around his head, hair all over the place, looking like a bear. (Not that the people in our band looked much different from him in those days.)

I said, "Did you hear what we had to say?"

"Yeah, man."

I kept going. "Well, what do you think of it?"

He was skeptical. "The only way you're going to change this society is to kick the ——— out of it," he answered. The students crowded around to see the conflagration! The intimidation was fierce. It was at that moment I had to count on the Lord standing by me and giving me an answer.

I said, "Did it ever occur to you that when you've kicked the ——— out of people you still have the same basic raw material? Don't you see that you can relabel the ———, then restack it into another political configuration, but you're still left with the same basic raw material? The problem isn't the system. It's the people. And Jesus came to transform people!"

"Wow, man, heavy," he said.

The truth God gave me to speak that day holds just as firm in this decade as it did then. New economic policy, welfare reform, a change of administration, intensified educational systems, more advanced technology—none of these human efforts or structures has the transforming power of the gospel we are privileged to proclaim.

In the last half of the nineteenth century, thanks to Charles Darwin and a fascination with evolution and the upward mobility of humanity, many held a blind optimism that our race would become more and more moral through education. Now, a hundred years later, what do we have? Better educated and more skillful criminals. Education hasn't transformed and never will transform society. Human achievement in and of itself is powerless to change the world morally and spiritually.

In his letter to the Philippian Christians, Paul is excited about the spread of the good news. He says, "I want you to know, brethren, that what has happened to me has really served to advance the gospel, so that it has become known throughout the whole praetorian guard and to all the rest that my imprisonment is for Christ" (Phil. 1:12–13).

The Roman praetorian guard was no insignificant band of soldiers. They were the Imperial Guard, 10,000 hand-picked men chosen to protect the emperor and to carry out other specified tasks. In the United States we have a similar though much smaller group of soldiers called "The Old Guard," based in Northern Virginia near the hub of power and ceremony. They're a spit-polish honor group, but no more select than the praetorian guard, who apparently were given the responsibility for Paul's security throughout the several years of his house arrest while awaiting trial in Rome.

Acts 28:20 implies that Paul was actually chained to one of these guards night and day to prevent any attempt at escape. Yet even in such undesirable circumstances, he spread the Word. Philippians ends with a strong testimony to his silent and verbal preaching. As Paul is saying good-bye, he writes, "All the saints greet you, especially those of Caesar's household" (4:22). Some of the Romans who came in contact with Paul had become believers—saints—under his influence.

In Romans 1:15 and 16, Paul forthrightly states his feelings about the privilege and responsibility of preaching: "I am eager to preach the gospel to you . . . For I am not ashamed of the gospel: it is the power of God for salvation to every one who has faith." Paul was consumed with a passion for spreading the Word.

Back in Philippians 1, he goes so far as to admit that the gospel is sometimes preached from bad motives: "Some indeed preach Christ from envy and rivalry, but others from good will. The latter do it out of love . . . the former proclaim Christ out of partisanship, not sincerely" (vv. 15–17). Paul acknowledges reality and then betrays his exaggerated allegiance to the gospel by saying, "Whether in pretense or in truth, Christ is proclaimed; and in that I rejoice" (v. 18).

Evidently, since the beginning of church history people have been preaching Christ as a means of promoting some underlying selfish ambition. Let's face it: Some publishers produce and market Bibles only because there's money in it. Some Bible-thumping preachers only want to build up their empires so they look better than the next preacher. Elsewhere, in 2 Corinthians 2:17 ("For we are not, like so many, peddlers of God's word"), Paul raises questions about this practice; but ultimately he still concedes the value of any proclamation of God's truth.

I'll never forget going back to England to hear my old pastor preach his farewell sermon. He was eighty-four years old! He held up the Bible and forcefully said, "This is God's infallible Word; when you disagree with it, you are wrong!" This is the Word I was given to preach at my ordination; to preach with the conviction of Paul—because it's the transforming truth and life and hope that the world is desperate to hear.

Ever since then I've had a "reverend" in front of my name; this gives me a special responsibility to preach. But that title isn't a biblical one, and every citizen of heaven, every saint, has the delightful opportunity to spread the Word.

One evening several years ago I met a derelict on the street. He caught my attention and said he needed a few dollars, as his check hadn't come through. I wasn't about to give him cash so I asked if I could buy him a meal. "Yes," he said, "I want chicken wings." So I drove him to the place he suggested.

Now at this point I must admit that I did something thoughtless and foolish. I went into the restaurant, placed the order, and waited the ten minutes for those wings to fry, while I left this stranger out in the car alone with my wife! When I came back out, bless her heart, she was sharing the gospel with him, introducing him to Jesus. That man got more than "chicken wings" that night—thanks to my faithful, wonderful wife!

Prayer and Peace

Like a Christian's proclamation of the gospel, our prayer life is both a privilege and a responsibility. The night before he died of drowning, Joseph Scriven wrote the song called "What a Friend We Have in Jesus." Remember the second line? "What a privilege to carry everything to God in prayer!"

Just stop and think about it for a minute. Through the miracle of prayer, you can transport your concern for anyone to anywhere.

I have two brothers who live in Australia, virtually as far away from Pittsburgh, Pennsylvania, as anyone can get. It's one of those countries that seems like the "end of the line" to us Americans. You don't go to Australia on your way to somewhere else; you have to have a reason to go there.

Despite the physical distance between my brothers and me, despite the seeming remoteness of their locale, I can in an instant flash a prayer signal on their behalf to God who has promised to respond—anywhere on or above this globe. "Lord, be with my brother." I say it and in a sense I'm with my brother in that moment. Any time of the day or night I'm only a prayer away from anywhere or anybody. Even more significantly, I'm only a prayer away from God himself.

Don't let anyone tell you that you need to be on your knees for this to happen. A praying Christian can always do two things at once. Just as you can be in love—or in pain—as you walk down the sidewalk, work at your desk, talk on the phone, listen to a sermon, or shave your whiskers, so you can pray as you do any of those things, or anything else, for that matter.

Philippians 4:6 says, "Have no anxiety about anything, but in everything by prayer and supplication with thanksgiving let your requests be made known to God." In 1 Thessalonians 5:17 Paul says it more succinctly: "Pray constantly" about everything.

I can share with my Lord the most common, ordinary concerns of my life. I don't have to wait for tragedy to strike before I call on him or before he hears me. We have a God, a king, who is concerned about how we respond to the weather, about the shopping we do, about our recreational life.

Our family had a dog named Shane. I used to go out walking and would often take him with me; he and God and I would go walking. If I had had an especially exhausting day, I would just repeat over and over again, "Lord, I am weary," all the way out our very long drive and back. Whatever I'm doing, I can—and do—lay my heart out before him knowing that he's not some figment of my imagination. He's as real as my dog Shane and infinitely more able to hear and understand my words and even my thoughts.

Anxiety?

A former landlady of mine had a plaque hung on her wall that read: "Why pray when you can worry?" There's humor in that motto only because that's how so many of us live. If we worry, if we hold on to our anxiety, we fool ourselves into thinking that we have a greater control over the outcome of events.

If we worry on our own behalf, we feel prepared to face the disaster we're convinced is about to befall us. If we worry over someone else, we assume our anxiety will reduce that of the other party. Listen to what Catherine Marshall wrote in her journal, which was published after her death as *A Closer Walk*: "Having laid my concern before the Father, I get the feeling that if I do not frequently return to it in my mind and keep 'worrying' it, much as a dog would a bone, then there certainly can be no chance of solving it. It's a feeling that it would actually be irresponsible or frivolous *not* to do this.

"I slip into the worry stance in spite of telling myself over and over that God is the problem-solver."

Because we can't see into the future, we tend to forget that God is just as much Lord over the future as he has been over the past and is over the present. The old cliché "Let go and let God" has a future, as well as a past, emphasis to it.

With Thanksgiving

Before we leave this subject of prayer, let's not forget the attitude with which God asks us to make our requests: "with thanksgiving."

When we're aware of what a great privilege our "open line" to God is, we'll thank him for such an amazing accessibility. Think about earthly heads of state. The Old Testament story of Esther tells of a time when even the queen could be executed for entering unbidden into the presence of her king. The very structure of a traditional fortress-palace is forbidding and seems to say, "Stay out; no admittance."

Yet God welcomes us warmly into his presence. The veil that separated us "commoners" from his habitation was supernaturally split apart the hour Jesus died. Every one of us is welcome to "enter his gates with thanksgiving, and his [inner] courts with praise!" (Ps. 100:4). He's only a prayer away!

As we enjoy this privilege of prayer—and every other privilege of our citizenship—over a period of time, our thanksgiving should have a cumulative quality to it. Most of us are like children in that we're concerned with what we're about to receive, taking for granted what we already *have* received. So let me tell you a little story that starts with the line:

Once Upon a Time

A man named Kurt slapped the bar on top of his alarm clock and stumbled out of bed. It was September 10, just another plain old day at the office, or so he expected.

But as he was standing in front of the picture window in the living room, putting on his coat, he noticed a stranger carrying a briefcase walking down the street. Now this was a quiet residential street in a small Midwestern town where everybody knew everybody, so Kurt watched this chap for a while as he was looking at house numbers and the names on the mailboxes.

When he came to Kurt's driveway, the man turned in, walked up the stone walk, climbed the brick steps, and rang the bell.

Curious, Kurt thought, especially when he opened the door and the stranger addressed him by name, handing him the leather briefcase in his left hand. "This gift is for you," the chap said—that's all he said—and he walked away, back down the street, much faster than he'd come.

For a brief second, Kurt wondered if this could be a bomb, but he opened it anyway and couldn't believe the sight: money. Bundles of large bills. He called after the stranger to thank him but the man just kept walking, faster and faster, and it seemed as if he just disappeared when he got to the end of the block.

Money. Kurt counted it out. One million dollars. He was not about to go to work on a day as extraordinary as this. In fact, he immediately wondered if he'd ever go back to the office again.

A year passed. September 10 rolled around again. Kurt slept late because later in the day he intended to celebrate the anniversary of his fortune. But about nine o'clock the doorbell rang. Kurt rushed down the stairs and opened the door and there stood the same stranger with another brief-case identical to the one delivered last year. The man even said exactly the same words, "This gift is for you, Kurt," before he turned and virtually ran down the street and out of sight.

Kurt was ecstatic. What had he done to deserve this second visit? Even before he opened the latches he was sure he knew what was inside and he wasn't disappointed. One million dollars.

On the third year, Kurt was up at 6 A.M. peering out the window looking for the man carrying the briefcase. And yes, he did arrive, walked right up to Kurt's driveway and hung a left, as Kurt had envisioned he would.

When he curled his fingers around the handle of that briefcase, Kurt said "Thank you so much," and he immediately closed the door and started counting the greenbacks. Just as he expected, one million big ones.

A fourth, fifth, and sixth year came and went, and each September 10 brought Kurt the same fortune. Each time Kurt felt just a little less grateful than the last.

A seventh, eighth, and ninth year. . . . On the tenth year, Kurt wanted to run an errand the morning of September 10, so he left a note asking the stranger if he'd just leave the package inside the garage, where he'd pick it up shortly, thank you very much. Sure enough, when Kurt got home, the briefcase was sitting there against the wall, waiting.

The gift arrived on schedule for twenty years in a row, until Kurt didn't even think much about saying thank you, and then on September 10 of the twenty-first year, the stranger arrived in town, right on time, but he walked down the sleepy street without stopping. He kept right on going, past Kurt's house to the end of the block, where he disappeared. Now Kurt was just as surprised at this action as he had been when he'd opened that very first briefcase.

He was angry. He'd been slighted. He had a few names to call the errant visitor who'd done him a terrible disservice. How dare he walk right by as if he didn't care.

As I see it, every day of our lives is a gift from God that is equivalent to Kurt's million dollars. Do we thank God, "This is the day which the LORD has made; let us rejoice and be glad in it" (Ps. 118:24)? Or do we just reach out, always expecting *more*, a "thank you" very evidently absent from our lips and thoughts?

Peace, Perfect Peace

If we do take advantage of the privilege of prayer, lifting up our petitions and potential worries with *thanksgiving*, Paul promises a result that is the envy of the world: "And the peace of God, which passes all understanding, will keep your hearts and your minds in Christ Jesus" (Phil. 4:7).

Hannah Whitall Smith said, "There are two things which are more utterly incompatible than even oil and water, and these two are trust and worry." She's right, but I'd like to change one word and say that *peace* and worry are utterly incompatible.

Jesus himself spoke directly to this issue of a Christian's privileged peace. John 16:33 (NIV) states, "I have told you these things, so that in me you may have peace. In the world you will have trouble. But take heart! I have overcome the world." Neither Jesus nor Paul is talking about a peace that has retreated from conflict. It has nothing to do with people hiding from the world, seeking a cocoon of security. It's a peace in the midst of warfare, and that's why it defies human understanding.

The peace that reigns in our hearts is ours because we have a trustworthy, all-powerful king who walks ahead of us into every day's battles. He has overcome the world. And that victory of his means peace for me.

3

A Responsible People

Citizenship. It grants us rights and privileges. But it includes another dimension: responsibilities.

So often the word *citizen* is preceded by an adjective—*good*. Boy Scouts who help elderly women across the street are "good citizens." Members of the Lions Club who help children with visual disabilities pride themselves in being "good citizens."

In this democracy, good citizens study the issues and then, well-informed, vote on election days. As the old saying goes, they "come to the aid of their party"—or their country, especially when it's under attack from hostile forces.

And so it is for us who are citizens of heaven. In his letter to the Philippians, Paul uses the Greek word that means "citizenship" a second time, and here the word is more closely connected to the responsibilities of Christians. A New Testament translation by William Beck presents the original nuances of Philippians 1:27: "But live as citizens worthy of the good news of Christ." The Revised Standard Version renders the verse, "Only let your manner of life be worthy of the gospel of Christ."

Prove to the World

Lifestyle is one of those new words so overused it seems as if it must have been around forever. But even though it's a term only recently coined, lifestyle is what Paul is talking about here. He's saying, "Listen, you guys. Being a citizen of heaven has something to do with your lifestyle. A good citizen of heaven has certain responsibilities."

Paul goes on to give a reason why Christians are to live exemplary lives: "So that, whether I come and see you or stay away, I will hear you are standing firm, one in spirit, and fighting side by side like one man for the faith in the good news. Don't let your enemies frighten you in any way. This is how you prove to them they will be destroyed and you will be saved, and this proof is from God" (vv. 27–28, Beck).

What's he saying? Our manner of life, our lifestyle, betrays our citizenship in heaven. Such citizenship will threaten people who aren't a part of God's kingdom; intuitively they sense that they're on the losing team. The more sensitive among them even understands that, in contrast to us, he's spiritually dead.

Using a different metaphor, Paul addresses this same issue in his letter to the Corinthians: "But thanks be to God, who in Christ always leads us in triumph, and through us spreads the fragrance of the knowledge of him everywhere. For we are the aroma of Christ to God among those who are being saved and among those who are perishing, to one a fragrance from death to death, to the other a fragrance from life to life" (2 Cor. 2:14–16).

It's not unreasonable for Paul to say that one fragrance might affect two people in opposite fashion. The stores today are full of a certain perfume that has been around for some years. Obviously its aroma is pleasing enough to prompt a steady stream of buyers to lay down their money in exchange for its scent. But I know one woman whose stomach starts churning when she takes a big whiff of that perfume. To some it may smell heavenly, but to her it smells like death.

Similarly, a typical American who has minced too many cloves of garlic will go to great lengths to try to get the smell off his or her hands. But in some cultures people actually wear garlic necklaces to ward off sickness. (The bulb does seem to have medicinal qualities.)

When I was a teenager, before I accepted Christ's offer of new life, I met a Christian who threatened the living daylights out of me. Although he was older than I, in his twenties, I was much cooler than he—more athletic and worldly wise. I was teaching him about dating, and I had him beat, hands down. Despite all that, he threatened me because his manner of life, which betrayed his heavenly citizenship, told me I was dead spiritually.

Working Out Our Salvation

Before I go on to discuss some of the responsibilities of citizens of heaven, let me clarify one point. There is no way any of us can earn his or her way into heaven. Some people misquote one phrase of Philippians 2:12: "Work out your own salvation with fear and trembling." They like to pull those words out of the context of everything else Paul teaches and the phrase becomes an island country, declaring its independence. Paul is certainly not saying here, "You have to work your way into heaven by being better and better."

In Philippians 3:3–6 Paul lists his own holier-than-thou credentials, but he speaks of them in terms of their worthlessness: "Put no confidence in the flesh," he says. And then he continues, "Though I myself have reason for confidence in the flesh also. If any other man thinks he has reason for confidence in the flesh, I have more: circumcised on the eighth day, of the people of Israel, of the tribe of Benjamin, a Hebrew born of Hebrews; as to the law a Pharisee, as to zeal a persecutor of the church, as to righteousness under the law blameless."

If modern Americans were to list the ways they thought they could impress God, their credentials would be worded differently: I serve on the church board, set aside four hours every week for volunteer work, give more than 10 percent of my gross income to good causes, read my Bible, and pray an hour a day. I live above the law. I do not cheat on my income taxes, and I am just as kind to my family as I am to strangers whom I'm trying to impress. Now that's an incredibly impressive list and about as impressive as Paul's was, considering his culture.

But further on in the same paragraph, Paul says, "I . . . count them as refuse, in order that I may gain Christ and be found in him, not having a righteousness of my own, based on law, but that which is through faith in Christ, the righteousness from God that depends on faith" (vv. 8–9).

He's saying, "No list of impressive claims achieves for you or me a relationship with God by which we can enter into the kingdom of heaven and earn the blessing of God." He uses very strong words to warn against people who preach that we are justified by works: "Look out for the dogs," he boldly writes (3:2).

For all of history—including the Old Testament, the New Testament and the intervening centuries since—the human race has been tempted to make religion and achievements of righteousness the means by which they enter a harmonious relationship with God. But Isaiah 64:6 says that, in contrast to who God is, our righteousness and our righteous activities are as filthy rags. In the presence of God, our religious activity makes us no more appropriately dressed than the bag ladies I've seen in Pittsburgh would be in the presence of England's queen.

If we are counted as righteous before God—and those of us who are citizens of heaven are seen as righteous—it's because God looks on us and sees that we're clothed in the righteousness of Jesus. Such righteousness comes through our faith in Christ, as a free gift from God. Paul repeatedly makes that clear, maybe nowhere more explicitly than in Romans 6:23: "For the wages of sin is death, but the *free gift* of God is eternal life in Christ Jesus our Lord" (italics added).

In Philippians 2:12 ("work out your own salvation"), Paul is simply saying that we who have received the gift of salvation, we who have become citizens of heaven, should be the best citizens we can be. He's saying, "If you have received this gift, you need to go out into the streets, shops, offices, and homes and put your gift—your grace—to work."

Actually, there's another clause in that sentence. It follows in verse 13: "Work out your own salvation with fear and trembling; for God is at work in you, both to will and to work for his good pleasure."

As is so often the case in Scripture, Paul presents a tension: It is God who does his work in me; it is I who must go out there and do God's work. Sadly enough, too often Christians live on one of the ends of that pole. At one extreme, some are laid-back, always waiting for God to *do* something. They say, "I've prayed about it and now I'm waiting for something to happen."

At the other extreme are the activists who jump headfirst into the task at hand, as if the fate of the world depended on them alone.

Paul says that life should not be lived at one end or the other; nor should we vacillate between the two extremes. Instead, both frames of mind should simultaneously influence us. We must choose to obey what God has commanded, but the only way we can begin to do that is if we believe that God is indwelling us and empowering us to will—or desire—and work for his "good pleasure."

In short, we've got to be taking our responsibilities seriously, working as if it all depends on us and yet at the same time praying as if it all depends on God. We know that he is our salvation—and our strength for the tasks he sets before us.

Ugly Weeds

Something fascinates me about Paul's train of thought in Philippians 2. He goes from "work out your own salvation" to a curious command. After such a great statement I'd expect Paul to command some magnanimous virtue: Give all you have to the poor. Or I'd expect him to prohibit some sin generally considered to be on the most heinous list: Cut out all the adultery, rape, bank robbery, violence—the "big" stuff.

Surely Paul thinks those actions should be called to a halt. But instead of mentioning any of these actions he chooses to continue his letter with a word about our mind-set and speech: "Do all things without grumbling or questioning, that you may be blameless and innocent, children of God without blemish in the midst of a crooked and perverse generation, among whom you shine as lights in the world, holding fast the word of life" (vv. 14–16). Paul says, "Quit being negative."

I've lived with adolescents long enough to know their standard mode of operation. These children whom you've raised from the cradle suddenly become world-class experts on what you may or may not do: "Oh, Mother, you aren't going out like *that*." "Oh, Dad, you can't wear *that* tie with *that* shirt. And those trousers, they are totally uncool. I'm not going to be seen with you looking like that."

A critical and negative mind-set is something we may expect, though not approve of, in teenagers. But too often we don't grow out of it. Adults carry it over and it becomes a lifelong pervading mind-set that can destroy us and those around us.

I clearly remember one particular flight I made to England some years ago simply because those seven airborne hours were made unbearably miserable by the couple sitting in front of me. They picked incessantly at their two kids. They complained repeatedly to the hostess. Then when she'd gone about her business, they kept on about all the faults and injustices of the airline, the airways, and life in general until I felt like getting out of my seat and informing them that they had ruined my entire trip.

When the prophet Isaiah relayed the story of God's call on his life, he said that he saw the Lord sitting upon a king's throne. At this sight, Isaiah's immediate reaction was, "Woe is me! . . . for I am a man of unclean lips" (Isa. 6:5). I expect Isaiah hadn't been a man who was accustomed to cursing and swearing and telling filthy stories. He was used to moving among Jerusalem's powerful and polite society. So my guess is that the uncleanness of his lips was more subtle and prompted by the negative attitude that creeps into our lives and takes over if we don't work to get rid of it.

A grumbling and complaining mind-set works a little like dandelions: Do nothing to curb their growth and they spread all across your lawn, even onto the neighbor's lawn. Soon the whole block is one big dandelion farm.

What's my advice? Simply ask God to help you see the dandelions for what they are—weeds that don't belong in your front yard. Next time a grumbling, complaining word escapes from your mouth, just dig it out by the roots and in its place plant a marigold or a crocus. As we cultivate positive words, we spread hope to a "crooked and perverse generation" that literally is dying in want of the good news of salvation.

Think on These Things

It's no secret that words are rooted in thoughts. So if we're to get rid of the dandelion words, we must follow Paul's admonitions as he starts to wind down his letter to the Philippians: "Finally, brethren, whatever is true, whatever is honorable, whatever is just, whatever is pure, whatever is lovely, whatever is gracious, if there is any excellence, if there is anything worthy of praise, think about these things" (4:8).

We live in a world that generally rejects what is true . . . honorable . . . just . . . pure. . . . That's simply not what the run of the mill is filling their minds with.

It's certainly not the list of criteria checked off by the producers of our entertainment media. The television shows, movies, books, magazines, even billboards are full of images and words that would make our ancestors swoon. In fact, we live in a society that has mangled the whole notion of purity.

One of Satan's tricks is to take positive words and twist them so that they're used negatively. One such word is *Puritan*. They were terrific people, righteous men and women who raised their children in righteousness. But nowadays, who on earth wants to be labeled as puritanical? Young women in high school go out and lose their virginity because they don't want to be labeled *pure*. Or sometimes those who are virgins go to great lengths to pretend that they're not.

And what about dwelling on *truth*? We live in a world that is so used to dealing in untruths or half-truths that we go around listening for the hidden agenda in people's conversations. Why? Because we don't believe that what they say is what they mean. When you suspect that everyone is out to promote the advancement of number one—even though few people come right out and admit it—and you begin playing the same game, you start layering mistrust and untruths and "white" lies into a giant club sandwich which always leads to acute indigestion.

Dealing in truth is a responsibility that can be wrapped in many packages. Sometimes it means facing the truth about ourselves. One morning I sat in a restaurant and had breakfast with a successful businessman who thought he had it all together. But I saw things differently and I told him that his wife and young daughter were leaving him because of his drinking.

"I don't have a drinking problem," he said.

I replied, "Terrific. Then all you have to do to keep your wife and daughter, your family, is to quit drinking. And if alcohol isn't a problem for you, then that one demand your wife is making should be a real easy one for you to meet. I mean, nobody's saying you have to go to AA or to a detox center. You just have to quit—which shouldn't be difficult, *since you don't have a problem.*"

At that, he looked at me sort of strangely because, of course, he did have a severe case of denial. He wasn't dealing with the truth as Paul commands.

Paul also says we're to think about what is *gracious.* But negative and vengeful thoughts seem to make for better movie scripts to play through our minds. So we spend our waking moments thinking about the person who let us down, the slight someone gave us, the one-line comeback we'll throw out the next time so-and-so says such-and-such to us.

Satan delights in fueling the flames of our pain. If he can succeed in doing that, he knows our minds will be too occupied to contribute any positive influence in the kingdom of heaven.

The Original Positive Thinker

Paul's life was not conditioned by people's response to him. His positive outlook is obvious a few verses later in Philippians, when he talks of his own life. He's no longer just exhorting readers to think about praiseworthy and wholesome things. He's saying that he practices what he preaches: "I have learned, in whatever state I am, to be content. I know how to be abased, and I know how to abound; in any and all circumstances I have learned the

secret of facing plenty and hunger, abundance and want"
(4:11–12).

By his example Paul is saying that we can and should
have a positive outlook both in season—when everything
is going well and all our friends are faithful and we have
plenty to eat and see the silver lining—as well as out of season—when nothing is going right and Judas has just betrayed us and our cupboard is bare.

At first glance you might think that everyone knows how
to handle the plenty Christ often provides. And yet I can tell
you that many people who succeed end up feeling guilty
about their success; people who have plenty feel guilty
about their resources. This was especially true in the late
sixties and early seventies; wealthy people lived in shame
of their success.

But nowhere in Paul's writings do you find him ever feeling guilty about the great education he had. Nowhere does
he express guilt over the fact that fellow Christians were
good to him.

He knew how to abound, and yet he knew how to be content in hardship. He wrote an amazing passage in 2 Corinthians 6:8–10: "We are treated as impostors, and yet are true;
as unknown, and yet well known; as dying, and behold we
live; as punished, and yet not killed; as sorrowful, yet always rejoicing; as poor, yet making many rich; as having
nothing, and yet possessing everything."

For Paul, being in want was not defeat and having plenty
was not necessarily success. To him rejection by other people was not necessarily disastrous, and acceptance or ac-
claim did not automatically mean that he was A-OK. In his
eyes, success and failure were not measured by secular
standards of wealth, honor, power, or position, and that's
why he could maintain an even keel no matter what his
physical state.

Beyond Contentment

In his Philippian letter Paul repeatedly uses a word even stronger than *contentment*; he refers to his own rejoicing and he speaks a strong command to his readers: "Rejoice in the Lord always; again I will say, Rejoice" (4:4).

Now there's no need to command something when it naturally springs forth. I've been through this with my daughters, in many regards, but especially with the "magic" words, "please," "thank you," and "you're welcome." Those words seem to give young children paralysis of the jaw, just as the command that they're to share seems to give them paralysis of the hands. *Please* just doesn't naturally spill forth from a four-year-old's mouth; neither does rejoicing for us when problems are mounting up. Yet in the presence of problems, pain, or grief, we are *commanded* to rejoice.

The most painful experience I've ever faced was the loss of our son, Jonathan, who died just hours before his birth. Though I never held him squirming in my arms, he was ours. He belonged to us just as much as our three lively girls.

Kathie and I left for the hospital in the evening, and I set the girls down and said, "When Daddy comes back home tomorrow, we will have a little baby." We didn't know whether it would be a boy or girl, but that was OK with the girls. They just wanted a real live baby to hug and rock and fuss with—instead of a doll.

But my heart just broke the next morning when I had to tell them that our baby boy had died. I had to help them carry their grief. I had to support my wife who was in the hospital and not well for several days. I felt the loss of a special dream—having a son. I loved my daughters, but I'd grown up with three brothers and had longed for the day when I would have a son; I'd teach him how to play soccer and take him fishing with me. We all had to live through the terrible pain of loss, yet throughout that ordeal we consciously chose to praise God and rejoice in him.

That attitude did not remove the loss, but it did change our focus; we didn't come out of that experience all bent and warped, angry at God for taking our boy; or angry at the doctor, though we thought the death might have been prevented; or angry at ourselves, because we hadn't pressured the doctor. We didn't deny our loss. We didn't rejoice in losing a child; we simply turned our eyes on Jesus and rejoiced in him.

Terrific!

Every culture has its own standard polite greeting. Ours, of course, is "How are you?"

Generally, the polite response is short and positive, simply acknowledging the kindness of someone acknowledging our existence. My standard answer to that question is "Terrific." I didn't realize just how often I said it until my secretary went out and bought me a mug that has "I am terrific" printed on the side of it.

When I stopped and thought about that almost unconscious reply, I decided that it's not a half-truth. To me, *terrific* looks like Italian dressing; it's the oil of gladness mixed with the vinegar of sorrow. There are things that make me glad, and there are things that make me sad. Life is never a ten, and yet it's never a zero. The oil and the vinegar are always shaken together and the taste is terrific.

How can I honestly say that? Again, I've learned to rejoice. There's a popular little chorus based on Philippians 4:4 that we like to sing as a round: "Rejoice in the Lord always, and again I say, Rejoice." It's easy to sing the little ditty without much thought to the power of the words, which are as magic as "please" and "thank you."

Fixing Our Eyes on Jesus

The more I write about this Christian responsibility to live a life that's filled with the joy and peace of the Lord, the more excited I get. But suddenly I've stepped back and realized that this emphasis on the positive outlook might have the opposite, depressing, effect on someone who didn't understand an underlying principle: These responsibilities are not something we must simply force ourselves to do. All we must force ourselves to do is look to Jesus; if we keep our eyes on him, the responsibilities—the lifestyle worthy of the gospel—becomes a part of who we are.

I've taken no surveys, but there's one verse in Philippians that I'm sure must be Paul's most quoted sentence: "I can do all things through Christ which strengtheneth me" (4:13 KJV). It's a verse many people like to claim as their motto for life.

Paul wrote this of himself—in the first person; then a few verses later he makes an equally strong statement with regard to the Philippian Christians. Speaking in the second person, he said: "My God will supply every need of yours according to his riches in glory in Christ Jesus" (4:19). Any Christian can accomplish anything God requires of him or her because God provides the strength, because God meets the need.

Do you want to be a better citizen of heaven? Jesus Christ is the answer. Writing to the church in Corinth, Paul said, "We all, with unveiled face, beholding the glory of the Lord, are being changed into his likeness" (2 Cor. 3:18). As we look to Jesus, we begin to reflect who he is. His righteousness, his characteristics, his strength become ours. We can sense it within our spirits, and others can see it in us as they look at us. In Philippians 2:15—right after Paul exhorts his friends to cut out the grumbling and complaining—he gives a reason why they should have a positive spirit: "That you may be blameless and innocent, children of God without blemish in the midst of a crooked and perverse generation, among whom you shine as lights in the world." We are lights in a dark world.

Does the image sound familiar? Jesus spoke of people as lights; in John 9:5 he says that he is the light of the world, and in Matthew 5:14 and 16, he says that *we* "are the light of the world. A city set on a hill cannot be hid. . . . Let your light so shine before men, that they may see your good works and give glory to your Father."

How can Jesus, the light of the world, say that we are the light of the world? Because he lives in us! Because we radiate and reflect who he is.

The night before Jesus died he used another metaphor to describe the process by which the goodness of God becomes ours. He said, "I am the true vine. . . . As the branch cannot bear fruit by itself, unless it abides in the vine, neither can you, unless you abide in me. I am the vine, you are the branches. He who abides in me, and I in him, he it is that bears much fruit, for apart from me you can do nothing" (John 15:1, 4, 5).

This image used by Jesus also shows up in Paul's letter to the Philippians. Paul prayed that the Christians might be "filled with the fruits of righteousness which come through Jesus Christ, to the glory and praise of God" (1:11).

It is Jesus' light that we radiate and reflect; it is Jesus' fruit that we grow.

A friend of mine in England tells a rather remarkable story of two young brothers who, when they were bad, were sent to their bedroom without tea. My mother used to punish me that way when I was young. Tea, in this British context, is really what Americans would call an after-school snack—a piece of cake or some bread with jam. Being sent to your room without your tea was a traumatic experience. After a long day at school you were hungry and felt as if you deserved something to eat before dinner.

But these two brothers didn't seem to mind this punishment as much as I did because they had a secret escape. They went to their room, closed the door, and climbed out the window into the branches of a tree that grew beside the house. They climbed down the tree and ran into a nearby shed, where they played and ate the snacks they'd squirreled away for such a day as this.

Their plans worked for quite some time, but there came an awful day when their father announced that he was going to cut down the tree. It had grown too big, too close to the house. It blocked too much light from the kitchen windows. The leaves were a nuisance to rake in the fall, and, besides, it hadn't produced any fruit in years. It had no redeeming qualities and it was time for it to go.

These boys were horrified and quickly devised a scheme to save the tree. They pooled their pocket money and on their way home from school bought a big bag of bright red California apples. They climbed out the window and painstakingly tied the apples to the branches of that tree so their father would have a change of heart.

Well, their fruit wasn't discovered until the next morning at breakfast when the mother called the father to the window and said, "Look at this. Isn't this amazing?"

The father was truly impressed with the crop of red apples. "That really is amazing," he said, "considering that it's a pear tree."

Now you and I know that pear trees must produce pears, not apples. And citizens of heaven, branches of Jesus' vine, will produce fruit after the likeness of the life of Christ—as they turn their eyes on him and allow the things of this life to fade away.

The New International Version gives a great rendition of Hebrews 12:2: "Let us fix our eyes on Jesus." That's the only way we're going to produce "Jesus fruit."

4

Relating to Other Citizens

As citizens of an earthly country, our responsibilities might be categorized into two groups: We have some responsibility for ourselves—to earn a living, to pay the taxes we owe, to keep our garbage picked up. But we also have a responsibility to and for the community and the nation as a whole.

I can remember, for example, the rationing in World War II Britain. Everyone was asked to buckle down and tighten up for the sake of the common cause—surviving the enemy's assault and fighting back to defeat them. Rationing was simply part of our responsibility to the nation.

So far we've looked at a Christian's responsibility to have a positive and "clean" lifestyle. But now let's turn to a second group of responsibilities—those we have toward our fellow men and women, especially our fellow citizens of heaven.

We're Not Islands

In the late sixties Simon and Garfunkel sang a song that referred to people as "rocks" and "islands." It went on to describe a person who was impervious to the pain of those around him.

The metaphor wasn't a new one. In 1623 the English poet John Donne had used a similar image; but his sentiments were the opposite of those in the twentieth-century song. Donne said, "No man is an island, entire of itself; every man is a piece of the continent, a part of the main; if a clod be washed away by the sea, Europe is the less."

Going back further, to the first century, we see that Paul also had something to say about people, particularly Christians, being "a part of the main." This theme appears again and again throughout Philippians.

Right away in the first chapter of this letter, Paul speaks of the "partnership in the gospel" (v. 5); he calls his correspondents "partakers with me of grace, both in my imprisonment and in the defense and confirmation of the gospel" (v. 7); he admonishes them to "stand firm in one spirit, with one mind striving side by side" (v. 27).

Paul sees the church as a fellowship of citizens who work *together* for a cause, who fight together with the camaraderie of army buddies. The kingdom of heaven is not meant to be a loose confederation of island individuals but a unified group committed to the welfare of each other under the direction of the Lord Jesus Christ.

To use yet another image, a surgeon friend of mine once commented that the only cell in the human body that does its own thing is the cancer cell. It's on its own timetable; everything it does is in disharmony with the rest of the body; and ultimately it destroys everything in its path.

Large pockets of the contemporary American church seem to have a different view from Paul of what the kingdom of God is all about. They like to sit in a pew—or in their living rooms—and watch as someone on a platform sings or prays or preaches. The church becomes like a movie theater where a performance helps an audience temporarily escape the rest of the world. People come and sit, expecting a certain amount of privacy and anonymity while God encourages them through the preacher.

Just as the United States is becoming a nation of armchair athletes, it's becoming a nation of pew polishers. I'm reminded of that description of an American football game: twenty-two men out on the field in desperate need of a rest and 50,000 people up in the stadium in desperate need of exercise. In a similar way, in too many churches the pastor and a small band of helpers are exhausted while most of the congregation sits and takes it all in.

That's not what God has in mind for his kingdom on earth. We are to join together in intimate fellowship, what the Bible calls *koinonia*, where we can learn to share ourselves, growing more and more accountable to and vulnerable with one another.

Friends Indeed

In his letter to the Philippians, Paul seems to have had fellowship and mutual concern on his mind for a good reason. Let's look at part of his closing remarks to these Christians:

"Yet it was kind of you to share my trouble. And you Philippians yourselves know that in the beginning of the gospel, when I left Macedonia, no church entered into partnership with me in giving and receiving except you only; for even in Thessalonica you sent me help once and again. Not that I seek the gift; but I seek the fruit which increases to your credit. I have received full payment, and more; I am filled, having received from Epaphroditus the gifts you sent, a fragrant offering, a sacrifice acceptable and pleasing to God" (4:14–18).

Repeatedly, when Paul was in need, the Philippian church had sent him money, without any appeal from Paul himself. The direct mail campaign, the toll-free telephone line—just call us with your pledge—the every-member canvass, weren't part of the early church system. Actually, 2 Corinthians 11 says Paul refused money from the Corinthian church, because he didn't want to be considered a phony, as previous preachers there had been. He wanted to preach the gospel with no strings attached, and he apparently felt that the gifts received from the Philippians were sent with pure motives; the givers wanted to share his burden.

At the same time, the Philippian church had sent him more than physical, monetary aid. Epaphroditus, one of their members, had traveled from Greece to Rome to help and support Paul in prison. Being under a sort of house arrest, it seems, he could probably receive guests freely. So for some time, this Epaphroditus was at Paul's side as a servant.

For Epaphroditus this was no small sacrifice, as Paul tells us in 2:25–28: "I have thought it necessary to send to you Epaphroditus my brother and fellow worker and fellow soldier, and your messenger and minister to my need, for he has been longing for you all, and has been distressed because you heard that he was ill. Indeed he was ill, near to death. But God had mercy on him, and not only on him but on me also, lest I should have sorrow upon sorrow. I am the more eager to send him, therefore, that you may rejoice at seeing him again, and that I may be less anxious." Paul is sending Epaphroditus, who has been sick unto death, back home so that his family and friends will see for themselves that he is in good health.

There's such a wonderful give-and-take in the relationship Paul has with his friends in Philippi. He had introduced them to the good news. In appreciation they had remained loyal to him through his hard times. Now he, out of concern for them, was sending back home the man they had sent to his aid. The love here is circular: Each party is making sacrifices for the well-being of the other. Each party is giving and in turn receiving help from the other. What does Paul call this? A "fellowship of suffering."

A Fellowship of Suffering

No, you may say, you don't want to think of this kingdom of God on earth as a fellowship of suffering saints. But our being citizens of heaven doesn't exempt us from pain in this life—only in the next. We all have one choice to make: Each of us can suffer with Christ or without him. And if the fellowship of citizens of heaven is functioning as God intends it to, no fellow citizen will suffer for long in the solitary company of God.

Listen to this: "For it has been granted to you that for the sake of Christ you should not only believe in him but also suffer for his sake, engaged in the same conflict which you saw and now hear to be mine" (Phil. 1:29–30). If the Philippians are to believe in Christ, they are called to suffer for and with Christ and with one another.

A few verses later Paul says that we are to have the mind of Christ (2:5), and a little further on he says that he wants to share in Christ's sufferings (3:10). If I think about that very long and seriously, it raises questions. Am I to stare at a crucifix and say, "Wasn't that painful?" Am I to push nails into my palms and cry out in pain? Am I to try to imagine what it would be like to take the sins of the world on myself? I think not, though some people have at times actually injured themselves physically for this very purpose.

Paul is willing to withstand ridicule, arrest, and beatings for the sake of speaking and living the gospel truth. But along with the physical pain, he wants to bear in his heart and mind the pain *Christ* bore in his heart and mind.

Sharing in Christ's Suffering

Before we can understand more thoroughly the fellowship of suffering we have with fellow citizens of heaven, we need to understand some of Christ's pain. What did Paul mean by saying he wanted to share in Christ's suffering?

In any of its forms—physical, emotional, spiritual, mental—suffering may seem hard for some of us to understand. It's one of those concepts so large and vague that it floats over us like a cloud we can't grasp.

It's clear the Lord Jesus emotionally felt the pain of people around him. He joined with them in a fellowship of suffering. Nowhere is this better portrayed than in John 11, when Jesus arrived in Bethany too late to attend the funeral of his friend Lazarus.

The man had been buried and the family was still deep in grief when Jesus arrived. When he met Lazarus's sisters and friends, says John, Jesus "was deeply moved in spirit and troubled; and he said, 'Where have you laid him?' They said to him, 'Lord, come and see.'" Then, says John, with no fanfare or apology, "Jesus wept" (vv. 33–35).

The onlookers' response to Jesus' tears was "See how he loved him!" (v. 36). But I see things differently. The end of the story, of course, is that Jesus walked to the tomb, cried, "Lazarus, come out" (v. 43), and then watched as eager hands, eventually including Lazarus's own, unwrapped the shroud. My guess is that Jesus and Lazarus slapped each other on the back and then ate dinner together. So I think that Jesus, knowing the day would end with a reunion feast, was probably not mourning the loss of Lazarus ("See how he loved him!"), but rather entering into the suffering of Lazarus's sisters, Mary and Martha, and his friends.

In looking forward to the day when Jesus would walk the earth, the Old Testament prophet Isaiah said he would be "a man of sorrows [or pains], and acquainted with grief [or sickness]" (53:3); one who "has borne our griefs [or sicknesses] and carried our sorrows [or pains]" (53:4).

Reach Out and Touch

It's virtually impossible to separate Jesus' healing ministry from a "fellowship of suffering." Jesus, God himself made human, certainly had the power to stand on the Mount of Olives or on the temple steps and pronounce healing of anyone within and beyond shouting distance. But no—time after time, he had personal conversations with and even touched the people he healed.

In those days lepers were an especially "unclean" lot, abandoned by their families, thrown out of their homes, left to beg for their own bread and live with their own kind. Touching a leper was such a violation of the customs of the day that lepers were obligated to cry out, "Unclean! Unclean!" when they walked down the street. This served as a warning against contamination, ceremonially and spiritually as much as physically. Luke 17:12 describes what was no doubt a typical scene: Jesus entered a village and "was met by ten lepers, who stood at a distance." They knew they weren't to get too close.

Yet Matthew relates an incredible interaction between Jesus and such an "unclean" man: "Behold, a leper came to him and knelt before him, saying, 'Lord, if you will, you can make me clean.' And he stretched out his hand and touched him, saying, 'I will; be clean'" (8:2–3). The risk of that touch speaks volumes to me. It's the foundation of a fellowship of suffering.

If Jesus had employed an advertising consultant, he might have beat Ma Bell to her slogan: Reach out and touch someone. After all, that should be the church's motto, not the phone company's.

Come and Dine

Let's imagine another day in Jesus' life—what could have happened as opposed to what did. He'd spent a long, hot day teaching and healing the sick. Matthew says that a crowd of thousands had been with him for three days, eating up his words and his wonders, but not much else.

Jesus assessed the situation and said to his disciples, "I have compassion on the crowd . . . and I am unwilling to send them away hungry, lest they faint on the way" (Matt. 15:32).

The solution to the problem eluded the disciples: They were out in the countryside; the crowd numbered 4,000 men, plus women and children; the food donations totaled seven loaves of bread and a few small fish, hardly enough to feed the "staff" alone.

Now here's where Jesus and the disciples could have changed the direction of the story. They could have sent everyone home with a cheery "be warmed and filled" blessing, turned toward their boat, set sail toward Magadan and then pulled out the precious loaves and fish—their own supper. It sounds to me like something most of us would do.

But Jesus' compassion prompted him to act. At his word the fish and seven loaves multiplied so that the food satisfied the hungry crowd, with seven baskets of leftovers to spare. Then, the text says, he and the disciples sailed away.

Jesus saw needs and met them, and as citizens of his kingdom we are called to take on his mind. The compassion that causes him to reach out to meet needs should prompt us to reach out; the sorrow that causes him pain should stimulate our own sensitivities.

Here and Now

In our culture I see groups of people we wouldn't dare call "unclean," yet we nevertheless shun them. Take, for instance, the unemployed. When people lose their jobs in America they become social "lepers." People who once worked for them, who curried favor with them, don't find the time to return phone calls. Even the friends they've made outside the workplace tend to step back. Maybe the friend's security is threatened; if lightning struck you, it could strike me. Maybe his respect erodes; if you'd played your cards right, this wouldn't have happened to you; couldn't you see the writing on the wall?

Sometimes such "leprosy" afflicts those who are divorced or widowed. The awareness of our own vulnerability (could

I be the next one who's deserted?) builds a wall that separates friends. Distrust is projected onto old cohorts: Will she make a play for my husband?

An article in *Today's Christian Woman* briefly told the story of a new widow who'd looked to her church for comfort and support. But there she'd found instead a group of wives who'd excluded her and said, "You're no longer one of us." That woman left the church—any church—and is it any wonder why?

Where was the healing touch, the listening ear, the nourishment? Whatever had become of the fellowship of suffering that Paul saw in the Philippian church? When Paul had been down and out, they'd stuck by him.

But I don't want to give only a negative example. Let me tell you about some incredible people in my church. One woman, whose own personal needs are overwhelming, takes in and cares for foster children. Her powerful, loving influence on those young and not-so-young lives is transforming. Sunday after Sunday I see them, sitting all lined up in a row across the church.

At one time, for one reason or another, there were two windows broken out of her house. And what happened? Another woman in the congregation came up to me and said, "I've made arrangements to have those windows replaced." Now I knew about the broken windows, but I didn't know that the fuel tank was empty for lack of money. On that count I was totally surprised when another parishioner called—a woman who was ill and struggling for her very life—to tell me that a check was in the mail, to pay for fuel oil for this family. I hadn't solicited either of these responses to need, but the fellowship of suffering citizens of heaven, temporarily residing in suburban Pittsburgh, came through on that family's behalf.

A Fellowship of Servants

Why do some people "come through" so often? Because they see themselves as a part of a fellowship of servants, ready to respond to and obey their Master-king, Jesus Christ. The word *servant* appears several times in Paul's Philippian letter, most notably in chapter two where Paul says, "Your attitude should be the same as that of Christ Jesus." Then Paul goes on to describe characteristics of Jesus' life as a servant: "Who, being in very nature God, did not consider equality with God something to be grasped, but made himself nothing, taking the very nature of a servant, being made in human likeness. And being found in appearance as a man, he humbled himself and became obedient to death" (2:5–8 NIV).

God as Servant

For the life of me I don't understand why anybody watches wrestling matches on television or worse yet why anybody would pay money and drive across town to see a professional match. A couple of hulks ridiculously dressed get out there, make ugly gestures to each other, and go at each other, stomping, twisting, locking. You're never sure whether it's real or fake. Victory is a matter of either brute force or a fix!

Even so, that's probably how we humans would have gone about rescuing a selfish, destructive race. If we were God all-powerful and set our mind to redeem a world that had gone wrong, we might well have tried either brute force or "a fix."

Notice I use the word *redeem*, not *reform*. Brute force alone, of course, can make people "reform" by toeing the line. I remember all too well, for example, being a camp counselor of junior high boys some years ago. I had to watch over seven or eight of them, and one lad absolutely refused to make his bed. Our dorm was competing against all the others for a prize given for the cleanest quarters—which necessarily required that every bed be made. I was young then, about twenty, but I was older and bigger than these kids. So this one boy and I had a showdown.

I said, "You will make your bed." He said, "I won't." I said, "You will." He said, "I won't." I took him by the hand and began to squeeze. I kept squeezing harder and harder until he was on his knees. Tears ran down his cheeks. Eventually he made his bed!

That, of course, is forced reformation, which has nothing to do with redemption. God doesn't reform with brute force; he redeems. The Creator took on the nature of a servant, laid aside the prerogative of his sovereignty and took on our human nature. He even died as a condemned man.

Sadly enough, we Christians tend to romanticize the cross. Women wear jeweled crosses around their necks; elaborate gold crosses grace our church altars. But the cross is really a grotesque method of criminal execution. It's as if women wore miniature hangman's nooses around their necks or we set electric chair replicas on our altars.

John provides a telling firsthand account of Jesus the servant, who insisted that he would wash the feet of his twelve apostles as they gathered for the Passover holiday supper. As you might imagine, washing the guests' dust-covered feet was the job of the most lowly person on hand, a person whose ego was at the low end of the scale—a servant.

John includes an interesting exchange between Jesus and Peter, who refused to allow Jesus to wash his feet. Peter said, "'Lord, do you wash my feet?' Jesus answered him, 'What I am doing you do not know now, but afterward you will understand.' Peter said to him, 'You shall never wash my feet'" (John 13:6–8).

Then Peter changed his mind and let Jesus serve him. At the end of the scene Jesus explained why he wanted to wash their feet. He said, "Do you know what I have done to you? You call me Teacher and Lord; and you are right, for so I am. If I then, your Lord and Teacher, have washed your feet, you also ought to wash one another's feet. For I have given you an example, that you also should do as I have done to you. Truly, truly, I say to you, a servant is not greater than his master; nor is he who is sent greater than he who sent him" (vv. 12–16).

Jesus wanted his disciples to follow his example: They were to honor each other and lift one another up by serving. More than that, he wanted them to know that he wasn't asking them to do something that he wasn't himself willing to do.

Passing On the Word

Paul wasn't present at the Last Supper, but Jesus' call to servanthood had obviously been well communicated to him. His letters to the church in Rome and Philippi start with salutations in which he refers to himself as a servant of Jesus. In 1 Corinthians 9:19 Paul refers to himself as a servant of his fellow earth travelers: "For though I am free from all men, I have made myself a slave to all, that I might win the more."

Then, as I've pointed out, Paul passes on to his readers Jesus' call to servanthood as he describes Jesus' life: "Your attitude should be the same as that of Christ Jesus" (Phil. 2:5 NIV). In Philippians 3:17 Paul also asks that his readers "join in imitating" himself—the servant.

The Philippians were already well-acquainted with the meaning of servanthood. The word isn't used to describe Epaphroditus, the man who'd left his home in Philippi to minister to Paul in prison, but everything said about him points to a servant-style figure: "fellow worker"; "fellow soldier"; "messenger, minister to my need"; one who "[risked] his life to complete your service to me" (2:25–30). Wedged in the middle of these descriptions of Epaphroditus is a command of Paul: "Honor such men."

Who, Me?

Most of us resist being servants. It's a dirty word in that we don't want to be slaves. We don't want to be treated ignobly. Servants are the "go-fors" who run around behind the scenes, making other people's lives more pleasant, other people's ministries more powerful. Most of us want to be the up-front person; we want the dignity of office; we want people to take notice of us.

We also want to be totally in control of our schedules. A servant doesn't have the option of telling the master that he just isn't available right now. I expect that Epaphroditus's availability was more useful to God than his ability; that's what servanthood is all about.

John the Baptist spoke like a servant when he said of Jesus, "He must increase, but I must decrease" (John 3:30). That's the spirit we're called to honor—and imitate.

Putting Others Ahead of Ourselves

Several years ago a friend and I were walking the floor of the annual convention for religious broadcasters held in a Washington, D.C., hotel. Many of the booths are sponsored by companies selling technical equipment to radio stations. Still others feature syndicated ministries trying to sell their radio or TV programs to local station managers.

You can't attend this convention for too long before noticing that it's crawling with religious celebrities presenting a bright, successful image of their work. So after walking up and down a few aisles my friend turned to me and said, "I would guess that there is more ego per square inch in this building right now than anywhere else in the world."

Being horrified at the thought and not wanting to believe that he might be right, I ventured, "The United States Senate might be just as bad." But once he'd said the words, I couldn't get the indictment out of my mind.

Now let me contrast that analysis of our culture with Philippians 2:3 and 4: "Do nothing from selfishness or conceit, but in humility count others better than yourselves. Let each of you look not only to his own interests, but also to the interests of others." And from there Paul goes right into the description of Jesus as the epitome of servanthood.

Nobody is asking anybody to play games and imagine that he or she is the most inferior among us. It's not a matter of "I am nothing and you are everything." The idea is that we're to reach out to meet the emotional and physical needs of others—with motives that aren't self-centered and full of conceit.

As Christians we're not to do our good works in the way many corporate foundations give grants. They love to display in glossy brochures how much they give away, and where it's given, because it's all a part of their public relations campaign. They want clients and consumers to think well of them and so they're tax-deductibly generous. No, we're not to do what we do for others so it will look good for ourselves. We're to be a team, always ready to work for the victory of the group and the sponsor rather than for ourselves.

I heard a great story from Tony Campolo, sociology professor at Eastern College in Pennsylvania, who was working with street kids in New York City one summer. These were the kind of inner-city kids who live and breathe basketball. But, as in every neighborhood, not all these guys were equally talented or practiced in basketball skills.

One teenager was obviously at the bottom of the roster. Tony observed the situation for a little while and then called the good players together. He referred to the absent, not-so-hot player and said, "Look, I want you to treat him as if he were a terrific basketball player. You know that you are much better than he is, but I want you to begin to count on him, begin to act as if he's really good, and tell him how great his game is."

This was kind of an experiment for Campolo and, sure enough, by the end of the summer that bottom-rung basketball player was the best on the block. The whole team had benefited from the encouragement the stronger brothers had given the weaker member. Now that's voluntary servanthood in action.

Redemption on a Small Scale

Of course, Jesus Christ is the one and only redeemer of human souls. But on another level, as we Christians imitate Christ's servant-style, we can redeem the dignity of those around us. Through an attitude of humility that says to other people, "You are worthy of my respect and encouragement and service," we can in some small way redeem them.

My former congregation included one of the finest surgeons in the country. Occasionally, he and I would go out to eat together, and we inevitably would run into someone whose flesh he had cut on the operating table.

I noticed this scenario several times; it always moved me deeply. He would greet a patient, saying, "Why, hello, Mrs. Smith." With all his power and dignity and prestige, he could just as well have said, "Why, hello, Molly." But no, he gave up that place of power and came to her as a servant showing respect. He laid aside the prerogatives due his position and in so doing transformed the sense of dignity that patient had.

If Jesus could lay aside his godly prerogatives, so much more legitimate than ours, why can't we do it for one another? God doesn't ask that we do this in our own power. In chapter two I said that God offers citizens of his kingdom the unique privilege of knowing who they are, of possessing a dignity and feeling of self-worth. It's when we have that sense of dignity within ourselves that we're able to let go of the prerogatives that come with any earthly place of honor or power—or superior talent or title or responsibility—and then empower others by seeing them as better than ourselves.

5

What a Fellowship

How do we respond when fellow Christians share in our suffering and become as servants to us, lifting us up, putting our needs above their own? Again Paul sets before us the Lord's way of *receiving* as well as giving.

A Fellowship of Gratitude and Appreciation

Philippians ends and begins with an expression of Paul's love and gratitude for the people who have empowered him by their faithfulness, generosity, and prayers. Philippians 4:1 refers to the Philippian Christians as "My brethren, whom I love and long for, my joy and crown . . . my beloved." And after an initial salutation, chapter one starts: "I thank my God in all my remembrance of you . . . thankful for your partnership in the gospel from the first day until now. . . . It is right for me to feel thus about you all, because I hold you in my heart. . . . I yearn for you all with the affection of Christ Jesus" (vv. 3–8).

These people had come through for Paul, and he felt compelled to express his appreciation and special concern for them.

Many people find it difficult to get the words "I care about you" out of their mouths or even from their pens, although it's sometimes easier to write than speak words of appreciation. Paul actually has the courage to write—and I trust he would have spoken the words if he could have seen his friends face to face—"I hold you in my heart." Then, even more staggering, he says, "I yearn for you all with the affection of Christ Jesus."

The Greek verb used here moves beyond feelings of the heart. The image goes deeper, to the stomach, where the butterflies flutter. The King James Version renders a more graphic translation: "I long after you all in the bowels of Jesus Christ." Throughout the New Testament, that's the deepest possible expression of caring; it's the compassion of Christ.

Somehow we're so afraid of those words, "I love you," or even of a modified version, "I love you in Christ." The male half of the world thinks it sounds too soft and sentimental, and the female half thinks it sounds too sexual. Yet our friends and families need to hear expressions of our care.

Maybe even your pastor needs to hear those words. Some time ago a young woman in my church sent me a lovely card. Inside she'd written a short note of appreciation and the first words on the page were "Dear John, I love you." Now the very next week this woman was marrying the man she loved romantically; this card had nothing to do with eros. Rather she went on to explain that she loved to see me standing in my pulpit, fighting for Jesus, speaking out his word boldly.

Is there anyone who inspires you by the way he or she fights for Jesus? Is there anyone who has encouraged you or your spouse or your children? Anyone who has gone out on a limb for you? Anyone who has been a servant to you? Stop and tell that person how much he or she means to you.

There's a saying that words are cheap. But it's only a half-truth. There's a powerful connection between deeds and words. Remember the old joke about the wife who's been married for decades? She's withering inside because it's been so long since she's heard her husband say, "I love you," and finally she musters the courage to ask him if he does. The old boy answers, "Of course I love you. I told you that when we married and if I'd changed my mind, I would have said so." Just as faith without works is dead, so works without words can be dead.

Having cheerleaders at athletic games is a uniquely American phenomenon. The first time I watched an American football game on television and saw these scantily clad women dancing on the sidelines during breaks, I actually turned to a friend and asked what on earth they were doing. It didn't look as if they were leading cheers, though he assured me they were.

We Christians need to be cheerleaders for one another. The last chapter of the Book of Acts gives in fact a wonderful little insight into a cheerleading party that encouraged Paul in his faith.

Paul is just arriving in Rome to face his trial. This is the last journey of his life and he's entering the city. Luke, his traveling companion, writes: "And the brethren there, when they heard of us, came as far as the Forum of Appius and Three Taverns to meet us. On seeing them Paul thanked God and took courage" (28:15). The support of the fellowship of believers gave Paul *courage*, which is obviously the root of the verb *encourage* and its opposite, *discourage*.

Such words and deeds of love and appreciation are what cement long-term relationships. But sadly, I see too many Christians who are like itinerant secular businessmen who keep moving on, moving up, leaving behind relationships that have nourished them through otherwise hungry times. They use people as rungs on a ladder; and they just keep climbing without looking back. So many Christians show no gratitude to the people who introduced them to Christ or who fed them the milk and then the meat of the Word. Instead, an arrogance grows, and the old relationships are abandoned for others that seem more advantageous.

If you read the Book of Acts and then Paul's various epistles, it's obvious that this mentality was not part of one particular friendship of special significance to Paul. On his first long missionary journey, the apostle had met a younger man named Timothy, who'd become a Christian under his ministry. Paul became a mentor to Timothy, and the young man later accompanied Paul on most of his journeys.

Although Paul actually penned the letter to the Philippians, he opens the correspondence by saying that the message also is from Timothy, who is with him at Rome. In 2:20–22, Paul points out Timothy's faithfulness: "I have no one like him, who will be genuinely anxious for your welfare. They all look after their own interests, not those of Jesus Christ. But Timothy's worth you know, how as a son with a father he has served with me in the gospel."

We get glimpses of Paul's long-term friendship with Timothy only through the writings of Paul, so we don't know for sure that Timothy verbally expressed his love and appreciation to Paul. But this high praise of Timothy by Paul surely indicates that Timothy hadn't abandoned an old relationship just because it was socially advantageous to do so. Two of Paul's letters to Timothy have been preserved for our edification, and especially the second one details Paul's fond gratitude for the younger man's service. Paul didn't speak highly of Timothy only behind his back.

A Fellowship of Risk Takers

Within the fellowship of believers we should be hearing encouraging word after encouraging word. Yet even though we want to help people feel good when they need to feel good, there are times when any of us can benefit from having someone love us enough to sit us down and tell us that we've wandered off course. We need friends who will love us enough to risk intervention.

We should never try to help people feel good about what is bad. We should never try to help people feel comfortable in their sinfulness. That's the kind of fellowship Paul saw as needed within the fellowship of believers at Philippi.

Odious and Soon-touchy

Apparently two women in the Philippian church were, shall we say, fussing at each other. Their names were Euodia and Syntyche, although evangelist Dwight L. Moody used to call them Odious and Soon-touchy. Paul writes, "I entreat Euodia and I entreat Syntyche to agree in the Lord. And I ask you also, true yokefellow, help these women, for they have labored side by side with me in the gospel together with Clement and the rest of my fellow workers, whose names are in the book of life" (4:2–3).

The sad thing about this story is that these bickering women were not just pew warmers—people who sat in the pew so the minister could minister. They were "fellow laborers" of Paul, servant Christians who'd been side by side in the trenches with him.

Unfortunately this still happens within the kingdom of God. Two people for years can give their all for the work of the Lord, then end up taking each other on and dividing a Christian community. Congregations split over the most petty issues. People become disgruntled and leave the church. When that kind of friction and discord comes into the church, the family machinery of Jesus Christ breaks down.

When dissension does creep into the body of Christ, we're called to risk intervention. I can just hear your response to that statement. *Me?* Get involved? I'm so busy and it would take so much of my time. You don't understand. They're screwed-up people anyway. Maybe it really is better if one of them leaves the church and goes somewhere else. Or you say, Hey, let those two fight. Just as long as the sparks don't fly over into my household.

Of course it's easier to stay in your own little corner in your own little group, but God never called us to a rocking-chair life. Jesus said, "Blessed are the peacemakers" (Matt. 5:9). Nobody is ever going to admire you and love you until you have risked your own comfort zone enough to intervene and say, "Hey, you're out of line here."

Of course you risk having them hate you; you risk having them call you a hypocrite; you risk your relationship with them. But didn't God risk that and more when he sent his Son to earth to restore between himself and humankind the relationship that had been broken off because of Adam's sin? And aren't we called to please God rather than men? In Galatians 1:10 Paul said, "If I were still pleasing men, I should not be a servant of Christ."

Confronting in Love

The risk of intervention often involves peacemaking, but sometimes the problem that needs to be confronted is not the sin of deliberate dissension. Sometimes it's just an irritable spirit.

I clearly recall an occasion when I was ill-tempered with Kathie, my wife. Our youngest daughter, Sarah, who was five years old at the time, had recently had a lesson at her Christian school on dealing with anger. She had learned a Bible verse, which she quietly quoted to me. Bless her little heart! She said, "Daddy, 'a soft answer turneth away wrath'" (Prov. 15:1 KJV).

I knew she was right, and I knew I was wrong! But I was so indignant. How could a five-year-old be correcting her minister father? I spoke briskly to her, trying to defend myself. "I'm not speaking angrily," I said. She became very quiet and I realized I had hurt her as well. Her subdued withdrawal got through to me. Here was the minister, who had

taught the Bible to his family, defending himself from having to respond to it, and in the process, wounding the faith
and trust of this dear little girl.

She had spoken the truth, and she had done so because
she loved her daddy and mommy. I quickly "repented" and
yielded to Sarah's telling me the truth in love. I said "sorry"
to Kathie and I said "sorry" to Sarah—and I said "sorry" to
the Lord.

I have also seen the power of the truth spoken in love in
my professional relationships with coworkers, as well as
with family, friends, and church members. I remember one
of my influential parishioners being so angry with me because she altogether disagreed with a very important decision I had made. I said to her, "I love you, and I know you
love me. We just have a radically different point of view on
this issue. Don't let this issue change our regard for one another." There was no easy resolution to our disagreement.
It went to the core of our different personalities. But at least
we could speak the truth in love. We both loved the Lord
Jesus and were committed to each other.

I have a man in my church who for several years was the
senior layman. He was masterful at confronting me with
hard truth about my shortcomings in a gentle but very firm
way. He had what in the old language used to be called "the
gift of ghostly (spiritual) counsel"—and he had the quiet
courage to confront me with it. I praise God for that man.
We need more like him.

Mostly we confront out of anger and indignation, or we
refuse to confront because of cowardice. We either explode
or freeze. Neither helps the other person. But when someone takes the time and the risk to tell a friend caringly the
truth face to face, God's power is turned loose.

You see, whenever we confront, our secret weapon is to
be the same as God's: love. We aren't to obliterate those
around us. Any correcting we do is not to sound like the old
television commercial that showed the man with seven tele-

phones on his desk. Into each one he was obnoxiously shouting orders to faceless, surely tormented people. We're to use God's Word to pierce someone's heart, not to chop off someone's head or cut out someone's tongue. God's truth may be used as a hammer to drive home God's love, but never as a hammer to drive home our own fierceness or our own purposes.

Paul told the Philippians that he was praying for them "that your love may abound more and more, with knowledge and all discernment, so that you may approve what is excellent, and may be pure and blameless for the day of Christ, filled with the fruits of righteousness which come through Jesus Christ, to the glory and praise of God" (1:9–11).

If love and marriage go together like a horse and carriage, so should love and discernment or *judgment*, which is the word used in the King James Version. Love is not all sentimentality, nor is it solely a matter of rational discernment. Jesus made an interesting statement, recorded in John 7:17 and 18: "If any man's will is to do his [God's] will, he shall know whether the teaching is from God or whether I am speaking on my own authority. He who speaks on his own authority seeks his own glory; but he who seeks the glory of him who sent him is true."

It's easy to manipulate circumstances for the sake of our own little world, so that we end up confronting others for our own glory. Or, at the other extreme, we may never confront anyone on any matter because we always want to play it safe. But if we're doing God's will and not seeking our own glory, our love will be a love based on intellectual and spiritual integrity, approving what is excellent.

Philippians 4:5 says, "Let all men know your forbearance." Tyndale translates it as "softness." Barclay uses the phrase "gracious gentleness." Actually, the Greeks understood the word to mean "justice," but something beyond a raw, hard-core justice. This justice had a strong and sure foundation but it allowed a person to choose not to press his or her advantage so as to become destructive to another person. It involved a choice, based on strength and knowledge, to deal with someone according to his or her need.

Ultimately, then, the word refers to sure justice sheathed in tenderness. Gentleness, though, not weakness. Forbearance, which has nothing to do with being a doormat. It involves relating with a soft front but from a firm and strong foundation; a tenderness that springs from strength rather than wishy-washiness.

In 1 Thessalonians 2:11, Paul says that he exhorted and encouraged and charged God's people "like a father with his children," or like a nurse with the children in her care. Paul was a spiritual powerhouse, and yet he lifted up those who were weaker with fatherly gentleness.

When people first meet my wife, I can imagine what some of them are thinking: Now, that chap got himself one lovely, gentle wife. Of course that's true; she's a very gentle woman. But at the same time, she has an iron core that is, frankly, stronger than the one in me. She is a cast iron fist in a velvet glove. She can punch a straight left and right to the solar plexus; she can get right to the center of a problem and blow someone away. But she does it so gently and caringly that there's no question about her motives and her love. In fact, people actually love it!

In 2 Timothy 1:7 Paul gives a wonderful summary: "God did not give us a spirit of timidity but a spirit of power and love and self-control"—or a sound mind.

God offers his children the courage to speak the truth with love and soundness, whether to fellow believers or to non-Christians. And that courage and power he gives is like that of a prancing stallion; there's a bit in his mouth and his movements are reined in, tightly controlled. This is the New Testament meaning of *meekness*. As that horse is sensitive to every move of his rider, we are to be sensitive to the Holy Spirit tenderly guiding us. And in the same way, under his directing, we Christians are to steer one another firmly but gently, when the need presents itself.

Vulnerability—a Mark of Maturity

We've talked at length about some of the responsibilities set before us as citizens of heaven—responsibilities for our attitudes and our relationships. I've presented a picture of life that's full of joy and yet hardship. Remember, life is one terrific Italian dressing, made of oil and vinegar. Some days that vinegar is poured on us by others, but some days we dump it on ourselves. Our humanity takes over and strains our relationships. Weeds get into our flowerbeds.

Paul addresses this issue with some especially encouraging words to the Philippians: "Not that I have already obtained this or am already perfect; but I press on to make it my own, because Christ Jesus has made me his own. Brethren, I do not consider that I have made it my own; but one thing I do, forgetting what lies behind and straining forward to what lies ahead, I press on toward the goal for the prize of the upward call of God in Christ Jesus. Let those of us who are *mature* be thus minded" (3:12–15, italics added).

Paul isn't saying that he has yet to obtain his salvation; no, he was absolutely convinced of his relationship with God (see Phil. 3:8). Rather Paul, the magnificent and exemplary apostle, was admitting that he wasn't perfect—and to the members of a church he'd founded. He was their hero. But he didn't want the Philippians to place him on some imaginary pedestal and think that he was claiming to be perfect.

Paul definitely disclaims that he already has a "resurrection body" and is already perfect (3:12). He is saying that, while God counts him as righteous because he has put his trust in Jesus Christ (3:8–9), not until he has died and has received his "resurrection body" will he literally be like the Lord Jesus.

That is exactly the teaching of the apostle John. "Beloved, we are God's children now; it does not yet appear what we shall be, but we know that when he appears we shall be like him, for we shall see him as he is" (1 John 3:2). There will come a day when all that God has credited to us in Jesus Christ will become an absolute reality in our experience. "We shall be like him."

But until then Paul says he presses on toward "the mark" (Phil. 3:14 KJV), and that mark or standard is the character of Jesus—to be like him.

Further, the ability to acknowledge our failures and short-comings, the apostle says, is a sign of maturity. "Let those of us who are *mature* be thus minded" (Phil. 3:15, italics added). The one thing Paul did not want to fall back into was the trap of pretending he was something he wasn't. He was finished with the hypocrisy of being a Pharisee. Living behind a facade of self-righteousness was an "immaturity" he had left behind when he gave his life to Christ (Phil. 3:8–9).

One of the most greatly needed ministries in the church, our schools, our homes, and the workplace is the ability to be vulnerable. Only the mature can be genuinely vulnerable. And how refreshing it is. It sets all who see it free from the bondage of "pretending." It allows us to share our deeper feelings and to ask help to make our unrealized dreams come true.

Sam Shoemaker, a great preacher in the middle years of this century, found vulnerability to be, on the one hand, the key to evangelize the disaffected, and, on the other, the doorway for churchgoers who were just "faking it" to get a hold on a genuine relationship to Christ. When great leaders like the apostle Paul or Sam Shoemaker are able to say, "I haven't got it made yet; I still have a long way to go!" and can talk about it openly, why on earth should the rest of us waste precious time and energy playing games? We aren't yet made perfect! Whom do we think we're kidding?

Recently a young man came into my office and apologized to me. He said, "I have failed you. I have failed my friends. I have failed God." We talked for a while and finally he prayed a very perceptive prayer: "Father, I thank you that I can fail with you." In other words, he said, "God, I know I don't have to play games with you. I don't have to pretend I'm something I'm not. I know you're the kind of father who will let me fail and lift me back to my feet again."

We have a God who removes our past failures from us "as far as the east is from the west" (Ps. 103:12). "Your sins and iniquities," he says, "I will remember . . . no more" (Heb. 10:17). Out of sight and out of mind!

Paul knew he wasn't perfect, but he also knew those sins were buried in the ocean depths of God's love. When he said he was "forgetting what lies behind and straining forward to what lies ahead," he was not referring to a little psychological trick. He was referring to gospel truth.

Paul was able to let go of the imperfections of yesterday and to press on like an athlete toward his goal of being like Christ. The key to this was Paul's vulnerability.

I believe "invulnerability" is behind today's cult of mediocrity in the church; and I think so for two reasons. First, when we're unwilling to be vulnerable, we become rigid, and the rigid man or woman is unable to look failure in the face. It's too threatening. Without an honest response to failure, a person's capacity to "move on" is extremely restricted. Denial is not only the problem of the alcoholic; it's the killer of the rigid, inflexible, invulnerable person. It's a prison that bars its inmates from coming to genuine repentance and so doesn't allow them to press forward into genuine righteousness. Thus mediocrity results.

Second, when people are afraid to fail, they protect themselves from any possibility of failure. The easiest way to ward off failure is to not press ourselves to excel, to avoid setting goals that are challenging and so pose the threat of failure. Thus to strive for excellence makes us vulnerable, just as being satisfied with the easily attained makes us invulnerable.

Herein lies the defeat and mediocrity of the "impossibility thinker." He refuses to be vulnerable, and the direct consequence is invulnerable mediocrity.

Paul's image of the athlete straining every muscle and tendon is all the more vivid for the serious Christian: "So run that you may obtain it [the winner's prize]" (1 Cor. 9:24).

When I was in school I ran cross-country. I was never the best on the team, but as long as you come in ahead of someone, you add points to your team's score. I gave it my best shot, grinding it out over those miles, uphill, down dale, through mud and slush.

There was one particular race I remember well. It was a wet, typically English winter day. I was right at the back of the pack, but I was determined to beat this chap with whom I was running neck and neck. He'd go ahead for a while, then I'd catch up and lead. Back and forth we went.

Toward the end of the race, I pressed toward the finish line with everything I had. I pushed past this chap and the people along the avenue cheered me on to victory. Unfortunately this terrific story ends with my finishing the race and falling to the ground vomiting. But such was the price I was willing to pay to give that race all I had!

This image of running the race appears as well in the Book of Hebrews. The author has just listed paragraph after paragraph of saints who are long dead. Hebrews 11 might in fact be called an Old Testament hall of fame: By faith Abel offered a sacrifice. By faith Noah built an ark. By faith Abraham offered Isaac. By faith Moses left Egypt.

At the end of this long list it says, "Therefore, since we are surrounded by so great a cloud of witnesses, let us also lay aside every weight, and sin which clings so closely, and let us run with perseverance the race that is set before us,

looking to Jesus the pioneer and perfecter of our faith"
(12:1–2).

We're running the race, our eyes fixed on Jesus, and we're
being cheered on to victory. By whom? Our fellow so-
journers, yes, but also by a great cloud of witnesses who
have lived in previous generations. The fellowship of saints
from the beginning of history to the current age is rooting
for us, reminding us that the strength to continue is ours in
Christ.

Paul returned to this image in his second letter to Timothy, written shortly before Paul's death. He had finally
been tried and he knew that his execution was near. He
said, "For I am already on the point of being sacrificed; the
time of my departure has come. I have fought the good
fight, I have finished the race, I have kept the faith. Henceforth there is laid up for me the crown of righteousness,
which the Lord, the righteous judge, will award to me on
that Day, and not only to me but also to all who have loved
his appearing" (4:6–8).

As Paul wound down this earthly leg of his journey, he
looked into the future with an overriding calmness. The
race, the battle, was over and his redeemer and king was
going to usher him into a new land. He rested in knowing
that Jesus had justified him. He knew he had given it his
best shot as a citizen of heaven. Now he looked forward to
the glorification of being made like Jesus.

That glorification, that prize, he assured Timothy, was
available to all "who have loved his appearing." That means
me. It means all citizens of heaven who've yearned to be
like Christ—in life and in death.

But remember where we began this section. Vulnerability is an essential ingredient of genuine maturity. So don't
be afraid to fail! "He who is in you is greater than he who
is in the world" (1 John 4:4). "You did not receive the spirit
of slavery to fall back into fear, but you have received the
spirit of sonship" (Rom. 8:15). "Do your best to present your-

self to God as one approved, a workman who has no need to be ashamed" (2 Tim. 2:15).

The Lord urges us on. His Holy Spirit courses through our personalities challenging us to be more like the Lord Jesus. The finish line is in sight. It's all worth the risk. Hallelujah!

6

To Live Is Christ, To Die Is Gain

No discussion of our citizenship in heaven would be complete without taking a look at that moment when the king decrees that your life—or mine—on this earth is over.

In a healthy way Paul looked forward to the hour of his death, and he openly shared these feelings with his friends in Philippi: "For to me to live is Christ," he wrote, "and to die is gain. If it is to be life in the flesh, that means fruitful labor for me. Yet which I shall choose I cannot tell. I am hard pressed between the two. My desire is to depart and be with Christ, for that is far better. But to remain in the flesh is more necessary on your account" (1:21–24). Paul goes on to say that the more he thinks about it, the more he sees the value of living longer. He looks forward to visiting Philippi again; he looks forward to his earthly tomorrow of continued labor for the gospel.

I've mourned the death of my own father and my own child; a girl I loved dearly died of a brain tumor at age twenty-two. I have grieved with my wife at the loss of two brothers. I have stood at the deathbed of many parishioners, offered words of comfort to even more sorrowing families. And every time death plucks someone from my small family circle, my large circle of friends, or my larger circle of acquaintances, I'm powerfully reminded of my own mortality. Whenever I conduct a funeral, I'm aware that every person attending the service is at least confronted fleetingly with his or her own death.

Around 1600 A.D., when the great poet and preacher John Donne lived in England, the church bell in town was always rung to spread the word of a local death. But the solemn gongs obviously gave no details, no answer to the big question, Who? The town merchants and especially the outlying farmers would find neighbors and passersby and inquire—for whom did the bell toll? Death is of great interest to us mortals—as long as it's someone else's demise and not our own.

Donne, the same man who wrote, "No man is an island," knew how interconnected our lives are. Having heard the church bell ringing, he wrote what has become one of his most famous lines: "Never send to know for whom the bell tolls; it tolls for thee." How true that is, especially within the fellowship of suffering saints.

But a day is ultimately coming when the bell tolls for me in the sense that I'm the one who is cold and stiff and breathless. Not one of us is going to ride this train forever. Barring the second coming of Jesus in our lifetime, every one of us is going to die. But our society doesn't take well to this notion.

Who, Me?

I don't like to watch television commercials. When they come on, I turn to another station and watch another program for a while. That's what a lot of folks do when confronted with death—they change channels! But I still see enough advertisements to identify what many of them are doing: They want to feed that lie we all want to believe— that we're not going to die.

In one ad a sober-looking husband shakes his head and says to his wife, "We've been kidding ourselves." From his tone you'd think he was talking about a stockbroker to whom he'd entrusted his lifelong savings. But no. He's talking about breakfast cereal. They're not eating as much fiber as they should be.

Eat this breakfast food, join this spa, swallow this pill and live forever. That's what the ads seem to be saying. Do this, and you can be like a god.

Something in all of us wishes we could believe that story, which is actually a lie not too far from the serpent's line to Eve: "[If you do] . . . you will not die . . . you will be like God" (Gen. 3:4–5). But reality always has a way of confronting us with truth. Birthdays keep coming around, and the older we get the more suspicious we are of every new ache or lingering cold.

Several years ago I spent a terrible morning going through an ugly, degrading lower GI examination. Whenever anyone has those tests the questions rise to the surface: What are they going to find? Will they discover cancer? What if I'm dying? Hey, I don't want to die yet!

Several things may be going on at a time like that. We may have listened to the commercials too long. But on one level those thoughts are justifiable. The gift of life God has given us is worth holding onto as long as God has work for us to do.

When our daughter Carrie Ann was three or four years of age and we were giving her elementary lessons about heaven, she looked up with big wide eyes and said, "Why can't I go now?" She wanted to be with Jesus, whom we talked so much about.

As devoted parents, our reaction was quite human and typical. Kathie and I decided to cool her little heels a bit. "God wants us to live out our lives here and complete all the good things he has planned for us to do," we told her. And one thing the Bible makes clear: At our death, our work on earth is done. We go around only once—in this world, that is.

We Go Around Once

Evidently it's becoming more and more fashionable to believe otherwise—to believe that we're going to come around to earth and have another shot at it. Belief in reincarnation, a teaching from Eastern religions, has infiltrated the Western mind-set, until books on the subject have landed on national best-seller lists.

It's easy to understand why the possibility of reincarnation would be intriguing to so many people. If they or others have "fouled up" this life, they might well hope for better days and years the next time around. If they know they're not ready to meet their maker, they might hope to be more responsible when they return as part of a future generation.

Some have the notion that reincarnation is more or less like evolution. Through a series of lives, we can grow more and more spiritually and morally fit so that eventually, when we're good enough, a death will usher us into heaven, or the Eastern "nirvana." Edgar Cayce, who's had great influence in this area, acknowledged Jesus' perfection and claimed that Jesus was the original Adam who was reincarnated thirty times before he was born of Mary in Bethlehem and lived that perfect life!

I see two problems, however, with this concept of reincarnation. First, if souls are just recycled, how do you account for the population explosion? The world population has more than doubled since 1950. Just try to imagine what that multiplication factor will mean in a few more generations, about the time our children's children become grandparents. If we were all getting better, wouldn't the world be less populated?

But a bigger or more important question than how do you account for additional life is, how do you account for continued depravity? I don't know anyone who is perfect. There's not one of us who is ready to be escorted into nirvana because he or she is so close to perfection. As saintly as the apostle Paul was, he readily admitted his own state: "Not that I . . . am already perfect." The imperfection of the best of us is what makes Jesus' perfect life, his death, and his resurrection so pivotal to our faith.

Hebrews 9:27 states, "It is appointed for men to die once." Shall I paraphrase the verse? Death is a once-in-a-lifetime experience. That verse continues with another phrase: "It is appointed for men to die once, *and after that comes judgment*" (italics added).

The Sheep and the Goats

I know many people, students especially, who are drawn to this evolutionary notion of moral and spiritual perfection through reincarnation because it doesn't call for a decisive day of judgment when God sorts the sheep from the goats, the wheat from the tares, the heavenbound from the hellbound. They carry an unhealthy denial of the finality of that last breath.

But Jesus told a different story, recorded in Luke 16. He contrasted the lives—more important, the eternal lives—of two men, a beggar named Lazarus and a second person called only "the rich man." Jesus quickly summarized their years on earth, then added that death eventually called a halt to both their daily routines.

Now their lives after their deaths were poles apart from each other—just as they had been before—but their positions of comfort had reversed. The rich man, who had lived as if he were the center of the universe, was called into account for his choices. The Revised Standard Version uses the words *torment* and *anguish* to describe his eternal plight. On the other hand, the beggar Lazarus was "carried by the angels to Abraham's bosom" (v. 22).

When the rich man appealed to Abraham for mercy, Abraham held a hard line and answered, "Between us and you a great chasm has been fixed, in order that those who would pass from here to you may not be able, and none may cross from there to us" (v. 26).

Once he'd crossed the River Jordan, as we say, the man who'd been so wealthy saw life through new lenses. He no longer saw through a glass darkly, but he saw the naked truth. And with this new perspective, he sent a proposal to Abraham: Could he please send Lazarus back to earth to warn the rich man's five brothers "lest they also come into this place of torment" (v. 28)?

But Abraham knew that wouldn't work and answered, "If they do not hear Moses and the prophets, neither will they be convinced if some one should rise from the dead" (v. 31).

What is Jesus, the great storyteller, saying? Exactly what the writer of Hebrews said: After death comes the judgment. I'm convinced that six seconds after someone dies without Jesus, that person would give everything he had ever owned for two or three seconds back here to change his answer to the great question: What have you done with Jesus?

At that moment of death, each of us will stand before the living God. Nobody will avoid him, and he will deal with us one at a time. If we're citizens of heaven, if we die looking to and trusting in Jesus, our Savior, we will go into the presence of God. As John 3:18 says, "He who believes in him [Jesus] is not condemned." But if we're not citizens of heaven, if we've rejected Jesus, our eternity will be spent in hell. John 3:18 goes on to say, "He who does not believe is condemned."

In Philippians 3, Paul talks about condemnation in direct contrast to citizenship in heaven: "For many, of whom I have often told you and now tell you even with tears, live as enemies of the cross of Christ. Their end is destruction, their god is the belly, and they glory in their shame, with minds set on earthly things. But our commonwealth is in heaven" (vv. 18–20). Even so, any condemnation is not because God desires it (2 Peter 3:9 says that he's not willing that any should perish), but because we have "loved darkness rather than light" (John 3:19).

William Law once commented that people "are not in hell because Father, Son and Holy Ghost are angry at them, and so cast them into punishment which their wrath contrived for them." Rather, he continued, people who end up in hell are like people who gouge their eyes out because the sun shines too brightly for them. As Shakespeare wrote in his play *Julius Caesar*, "Men at some time are masters of their fates."

While There's Life, There's Hope

Just as there are two ways to live—with Jesus or without him—there are two ways to die—with or without him and the hope he provides.

Svetlana Alliluyeva published in *Twenty Letters to a Friend* a descriptive account of the death of her father, Joseph Stalin, known for his tyrannical, ruthless rule over the Soviet people. It seems his death was as ugly as his life. Svetlana wrote:

At what seemed like the very last moment he suddenly opened his eyes and cast a glance over everyone in the room. It was a terrible glance, insane or perhaps angry and full of the fear of death and the unfamiliar faces of the doctors bent over him. The glance swept over everyone in a second. Then something incomprehensible and awesome happened that to this day I can't forget and don't understand. He suddenly lifted his left hand as though he were pointing to something above and bringing down a curse on us all. The gesture was incomprehensible and full of menace, and no one could say to whom or what it might be directed. The next moment, after a final effort, the spirit wrenched itself free of the flesh.

That was a death I'm glad I didn't have to witness, and any of us can only imagine what his torment was—and is. But the scenario didn't have to have such a bleak ending, even for someone whose life record was as black as Joseph Stalin's.

God's mercy, his offer of forgiveness and citizenship in heaven, endures to the last split second of our physical life. As Cicero said, "While there's life, there's hope."

Remember the story of the thief who died on the cross next to Jesus? He knew his hours were numbered, and in those last minutes, he turned to Jesus and got his faith in order. Jesus assured him that by the day's end he would be whisked away—into paradise.

I thank God there's always hope. But I get nervous when I listen to people who talk as if the thief on the cross was their patron saint. Oh yes, they believe that there's a finality about death and they believe in a subsequent judgment, but they're confident that they have firm control over their own future timetable. They're depending on having opportunity for a deathbed repentance. If it worked for the thief, they say, it can work for me. I'll live like the devil and die like a saint.

Now anyone who's waiting for that last opportunity is playing Russian roulette with his or her eternal soul. As a pastor I've consoled family after family mourning the death of their loved ones whose lives were snuffed out as quickly as a candle flame pinched between thumb and finger. I remember one woman in particular. While sitting next to her daughter at a luncheon, she quietly fell limp. The puzzled daughter thought her mother was resting her head on the daughter's shoulder, but actually she had died—without a moment's warning.

None of us, no matter what our age, knows what a day will bring. That's why Paul said, "Behold, *now* is the acceptable time; behold, *now* is the day of salvation" (2 Cor. 6:2, italics added).

Paul, No Stranger to Death

Paul knew how fragile life was. Long before his execution in Rome he'd had a chance to face the possibility of his own death. We've discussed a few instances when Paul's life was in danger because of the message he was preaching. But the New Testament mentions many more, including an incident in Jerusalem when Paul was dragged from the temple and would have been lynched if Roman soldiers hadn't stepped in and stopped the beating (Acts 21:30–32).

But Paul faced his own death again in several circumstances that we'd call "acts of God." As a prisoner on his way to Rome, the boat on which he was a passenger got caught in a hurricane. Acts 27:20 gives a commentary on his plight: "All hope of our being saved was at last abandoned."

A few weeks later, when the crippled ship had drifted within sight of land and the starving sailors had swum to the island shore, Paul tangled with yet another death threat: As he was gathering sticks to kindle a fire, he was bitten by a deadly poisonous snake.

Now Paul lived to tell the story, but having faced his own mortality, he knew that his own death in Christ was an event he would not fear. To the Philippians he could say that death was an advancement. And to the Corinthians he had written, "Death is swallowed up in victory. . . . O death, where is thy sting? . . . Thanks be to God, who gives us the victory through our Lord Jesus Christ" (1 Cor. 15:54–57).

The Holy Spirit clearly gave Paul the insight that death in Christ was not a curse to be feared. But I have a strong suspicion that the scene he had observed firsthand added some steel to his convictions.

Becoming Like Christ in Death

Paul had seen many people die. In his day, in his land, public execution was commonplace. Capital punishment was carried out frequently and not quietly and privately inside the walls of prisons. Political rebels and criminals alike were slowly tortured to death alongside well-traveled roadways as a reminder: Beware; your deeds will surely find you out. In Paul's day, critically ill people weren't rushed away in ambulances and cared for by professionals. Death struck close to home, where families watched over the process.

But the New Testament goes into detail about only one death Paul observed, and the details would have been hard to forget. Stephen had just preached a hard-hitting sermon to a large crowd of Jews in Jerusalem who became furious because he was pointing out their sin of resisting the Holy Spirit.

Acts 7:54–8:1 says, "Now when they heard these things . . . they ground their teeth against him. But he, full of the Holy Spirit, gazed into heaven and saw the glory of God, and Jesus standing at the right hand of God; and he said, 'Behold, I see the heavens opened, and the Son of man standing at the right hand of God.' But they cried out with a loud voice and stopped their ears and rushed together upon him. Then they cast him out of the city and stoned him; and the witnesses laid down their garments at the feet of a young man named Saul. And as they were stoning Stephen, he prayed, 'Lord Jesus, receive my spirit.' And he knelt down and cried with a loud voice, 'Lord, do not hold this sin against them.' And when he had said this, he fell asleep. *And Saul was consenting to his death*" (italics added).

The consenting Saul, of course, was the apostle Paul in his preconversion days.

What a contrast between this death and Joseph Stalin's. Stephen didn't bring down a curse; he wasn't angry at how the world had dealt with him, or how he had dealt with the world; he wasn't tortured with fear, challenging in anger the unseen world of the spirit.

But what similarities between Stephen's death and Jesus' own. Although Paul could very well have been in Jerusalem at the time of Jesus' crucifixion, there's nothing in the New Testament that gives us reason to believe Paul was an eyewitness to that event as he was to Stephen's martyrdom. But after Paul's conversion, as a new Christian, he'd have heard the disciples' firsthand accounts of Jesus' last phrases: "Father, forgive them; for they know not what they do" (Luke 23:34); "Father, into thy hands I commit my spirit!" (Luke 23:46).

Now there's a model for a death with dignity, and that's how Paul desired to die. In the middle of the Philippian letter he tells his friends that he wants to become like Jesus in his death (3:10).

Sweet Release

Although we Christians can and should value every day we're given by God, I see tragedy in the way some believers hang onto life with a desperation no less feverish than that of many pagans. They run from one healing service to another, obsessed with demands that God restore their health.

But both Jesus and Stephen were willing to release themselves into God's hands. In the hour of death, they trusted themselves to the One they knew to be in control. Do you remember a scene at Jesus' trial? Pilate, impressed with his position of authority, threatened Jesus: "Do you not know that I have power to release you, and power to crucify you?" (John 19:10). That kind of intimidation works on people who fear death and are desperate to hold on to life.

But Jesus came back with a challenge that proved his godly courage: "You would have no power over me unless it had been given you from above" (v. 11). He could let go of life because he knew the God who was—and is— stronger than death.

Stephen and the apostle Paul could face death because they knew where their citizenship was. Paul knew his name was written in the Book of Life; for him death meant being called home. It meant going to be with King Jesus!

I love the story behind the writing of an old gospel song, "It Is Well with My Soul." The author, Horatio Spafford, had lost his family when the ship they were on sank in the Atlantic Ocean. He grieved their loss as any husband and father would. But some time later he crossed the Atlantic by ship. When the captain pointed out the spot where the other ship had gone down, Spafford penned the words that Philip Bliss put to music:

When peace like a river attendeth my way,
When sorrows like sea billows roll;
Whatever my lot, Thou hast taught me to say,
It is well, it is well with my soul.

Though Satan should buffet, though trials should come,
Let this blest assurance control,
That Christ hath regarded my helpless estate,
And hath shed His own blood for my soul.

My sin—oh, the bliss of this glorious thought—
My sin, not in part, but the whole,
Is nailed to His cross and I bear it no more,
Praise the Lord, praise the Lord, O my soul.

And, Lord, haste the day when our faith shall be sight,
The clouds be rolled back as a scroll,
The trumpet shall sound and the Lord shall descend;
Even so it is well with my soul.

Spafford knew he was ready. If the ship he'd boarded had started taking on water right then and there, he would have faced death without fear.

That same assurance is mine—and can be yours. Remember, while there's life, there is the opportunity to turn your life over to Jesus the Savior.

A Prayer

Lord Jesus, when confronted with death we want to run in the opposite direction. But we acknowledge right now that our death is ever before us, for we don't know the hour when our time here will be over. With the apostle Paul, we want to be able to say that to live is Christ and to die is gain. We desire to become like Christ in his death and be able to say, "Father, into thy hands I commit my spirit," with full confidence that we will be welcomed into your kingdom of heaven. We come to you, Lord, casting ourselves on you and claiming your promise of mercy and grace. We believe, Lord. Help our unbelief. Amen.

7

Going Home

What will eternity be like for those who have died as citizens of heaven? That question has been on the minds of theologians, writers, poets, and dreamers for centuries.

Previously I mentioned the Old Testament hall of fame that's presented in Hebrews 11: By faith Abel offered a sacrifice, Noah built an ark, Moses left Egypt. . . . In the middle of this list, the writer inserts an interesting comment: "These all died in faith, not having received what was promised, but having seen it and greeted it from afar, and having acknowledged that they were strangers and exiles on the earth. For people who speak thus make it clear that they are seeking a homeland. If they had been thinking of that land from which they had gone out, they would have had opportunity to return. But as it is, they desire a better country, that is, a heavenly one. Therefore God is not ashamed to be called their God, for he has prepared for them a city" (11:13–16).

This first-century writer knew that saints from the beginning of time longed to go home to heaven. They knew they were foreigners on earth.

When circumstances here on earth seem especially bleak, imaginings of that future glory have kindled hope that has been transformed into strength, much as twigs are transformed into heat when they're lit with fire. The spirituals once sung by American slaves are full of heavenly images that helped a suffering people hold on as long as life held them to this earth: "Swing low, sweet chariot, coming for to carry me home"; "There are twelve gates to the city"; "I'll fly away."

More recent gospel song writers have sung the same tune: "I've got a mansion just over the hilltop"; "Beulah Land, sweet Beulah Land"; "When we all get to heaven." Even subdued Episcopalians join in when they sing, "Jerusalem the golden, with milk and honey blest."

Land Beyond Compare

Even so, that eternal place of beauty and security and, most important, of fellowship with God, our creator and redeemer and lover and king, is not simply a fairy-tale land manufactured by weak and weary pilgrims who needed a solace. We find out more about this place called heaven from the apostle John than we do from Paul.

In his last days of exile on the island of Patmos, John was given a vision of the future that allowed him to see inside the gates of heaven. In the Book of Revelation, John described a physical city decorated with ornate jewels and precious metals, even streets of gold. Until we see for ourselves, we won't know for sure whether or not the streets will be paved with gold as we know it. But one thing is sure: The heaven that God has prepared for the people of his kingdom is a place that is beyond any earthly scale of measurement.

Every four years when we watch the Olympic games, we eagerly wait for some bright young star to receive a judge's ten, the standard of perfection. In the 1984 Summer Olympics, Mary Lou Retton achieved what seemed the impossible. All the eagle-eye judges gave tens to her vaulting performance. In that event she was perfection personified.

What will heaven be like? Even more than perfection. Everything needed to fulfill our desires will be there and with such intensity, such quality and beauty, that it isn't measurable by our standards. If ten is a measure of perfection, heaven is unimaginably beyond that.

People who have had good marriages and who face the death of spouses are sometimes unsettled by Jesus' comment that in heaven there will be no marriage. But we mortals think this way only because of our blurred vision, only because we see through the glass darkly. Married people can't fathom a future world in which they will be utterly fulfilled without that exclusive relationship that has been so important to them.

A Heavenly Home

Whether or not we've had what we consider a "good" childhood or a happy adult life, most of us have a notion of what a perfect home would be like: love, security, laughter, plenty, rest, familiarity. In heaven, God's children will feel more at home than they ever did on earth. There's a kernel of truth in Cicero's remark: "I depart from life as from an inn, and not as from my home."

In John 14, Jesus himself says, "In my Father's house are many rooms"—many dwelling places. "If it were not so, would I have told you that I go to prepare a place for you? And when I go and prepare a place for you, I will come again and will take you to myself, that where I am you may be also" (vv. 2–3).

Jesus left this earth to go and prepare a place for each and every one of the citizens of his kingdom. In other words, each dwelling place will have a name on the door. My name will be carved on one door, yours on another. No one will feel as if he or she is temporarily living in a guest room, in a makeshift situation that doesn't quite feel like home.

Consider a familiar childhood scenario that shows what death is like to a Christian: Your family is visiting friends or relatives and the evening drags on until you grow sleepy, sleepier. You fall asleep on the couch or in someone else's bed. Then without your even knowing, your father picks you up and carries you to the car, drives home, then takes you up the stairs and tucks you into your own bed. When you wake up, it's morning, the sun is shining and you're snug under your own covers, hugging your own stuffed rabbit. So it will be when we die. We'll go to sleep here and the next morning wake up there—in that place Jesus has prepared for us, that place that will feel more like home than any home we've ever known.

With Him

Now heaven is a place, just as any home we've ever had was a place. But, as Cheryl Forbes says in her book *Catching Sight of God*, "heaven is unlike other places we know, for it exists outside of time. It isn't mere extravagance; it is merely God's home. Without God, heaven would cease to be: place and person are inseparable."

We will not go to heaven and there enjoy our solitude. We will go there and be in the very presence of God—Father, Son, and Spirit. Let me repeat Jesus' words about heaven: "That where I am you may be also." In *Grace Grows Best in Winter*, Margaret Clarkson says, "God has disclosed that His ultimate purpose for every Christian is nothing less than an eternity spent in His own presence."

When I dwell on that—being with Jesus himself and in a world where clocks do not tick away the hours, where there are only hellos and no goodbyes—I can say a hearty "amen" to Paul's sentiment in Philippians 1:23: "My desire is to depart and be with Christ, for that is far better" than life on earth. That doesn't mean Paul took matters into his own hands and changed his permanent residence. As long as God had work for Paul to do, Paul was willing to stay put.

A favorite writer of mine, C. S. Lewis, made a fascinating observation in *Mere Christianity*: "If you read history you will find that the Christians who did the most for the present world were precisely those who thought the most of the next. It is since Christians have largely ceased to think of the other world that they have become so ineffective in this."

That was obviously true in the case of Paul. He longed to go home and be with Jesus, but what he achieved before he left changed the history of the world—and my history as well.

With Him and Like Him

The words of Paul—"My desire is to depart and be with Christ"—and other Scriptures, including the words of Jesus to the thief on the cross, convince me that on our death our spirits are immediately transported to the heavenly dwelling awaiting us. All of us who walk with Jesus through the valley of death will be ushered into the presence of God. But then we will await yet another transformation: the resurrection of our bodies.

Paul refers to this in Philippians 3:20 and 21: "But our commonwealth is in heaven, and from it we await a Savior, the Lord Jesus Christ, who will change our lowly body to be like his glorious body, by the power which enables him even to subject all things to himself."

At some future moment—it could even be today—a victorious Jesus will crack like lightning through time and space and descend to earth, drawing history to a close.

In 1 Thessalonians Paul gives a more detailed account of that day: "But we would not have you ignorant, brethren, concerning those who are asleep, that you may not grieve as others do who have no hope. For since we believe that

Jesus died and rose again, even so, through Jesus, God will bring with him those who have fallen asleep. For this we declare to you by the word of the Lord, that we who are alive, who are left until the coming of the Lord, shall not precede those who have fallen asleep. For the Lord himself will descend from heaven with a cry of command, with the archangel's call, and with the sound of the trumpet of God. And the dead in Christ will rise first; then we who are alive, who are left, shall be caught up together with them in the clouds to meet the Lord in the air; and so we shall always be with the Lord. Therefore comfort one another with these words" (4:13–18).

On that day, all citizens of heaven, whether dead or alive, will receive bodies like that of Jesus. Our spirits will be clothed in new and glorious bodies. They will be ours forever, yet as the centuries click by we'll not see a wrinkle, spot, or blemish; we'll not feel an itch, an ache, or a pain.

In this life, there may be more than a little truth in the humorous saying, "After forty it's patch, patch, patch." I've hit the big fifty, and despite the healthy breakfast I may eat and the exercise regimen I may keep, I can tell you—my wife and my doctor can tell you—that my body is walking down the far side of the mountain. Physically, I've passed my peak. But in that future world there's going to be no such thing as "past his prime." Every one of us is going to be at his or her best—world without end, amen.

In that future world the ad men—here I'll let my imagination get away with me—won't need to camouflage reality with makeup and facades; they won't need to promote a lie—that we'll be young forever, that we'll never die, that we'll be godlike—because that will be the truth of the matter: We will be like Christ. Paul isn't the only New Testament writer to say this. John reiterates the point: "Beloved, we are God's children now; it does not yet appear what we shall be, but we know that when he appears we shall be like him, for we shall see him as he is" (1 John 3:2).

A Mystery

In yet another passage where Paul describes this resurrection morning, he says, "Lo! I tell you a mystery. . . . we shall all be changed. . . . For this perishable nature must put on the imperishable, and this mortal nature must put on immortality" (1 Cor. 15:51–53).

The *how* of this resurrection is indeed a mystery to me, but that incomprehension isn't an obstacle to my sure belief that my God can and will pull it off. The bodies of martyrs who've been torn limb from limb, of soldiers and civilians who've been burned to ashes, of children who've decayed to dust, all will rise intact and in perfect condition.

I can't begin to tell you how a Sunday morning church service appears without delay on a TV screen in a parish hall set up to accommodate an overflow crowd. If we ordinary human beings can do that—and even flash a church service up to a satellite and bounce it back so that it appears live on another continent—it's going to be no big deal for God, creator of the universe, to orchestrate the resurrection of the long dead.

Questions of *how* and *when* don't concern me nearly as much as the question *if*: If Jesus returned today, would we be ready? In Matthew 25:13 Jesus speaks of this future day with a word of warning: "Watch therefore, for you know neither the day nor the hour." Be ready, he says. Be ready.

Many Christians are thoroughly convinced that we are living through the last of the last days, and it may well be true. But a look at church history would show that watchers of the times have seen "clear" signs of the end in nearly every century since Jesus' ascension. Even first-century Christians thought that the days of the earth were numbered—on fingers and toes. Although the years since Jesus' promise that he will soon return (Rev. 22:20) seem long to us mortals, they are not long in God's view of time, where a day is like a thousand years and a thousand years like a day. However *soon* may be defined, the question is, Will you be ready to greet him with open arms as your long-awaited king?

Would you know the stance you'd take in the scene described by Paul in Philippians 2:10 and 11? Speaking of future events he said, ". . . that at the name of Jesus every knee should bow, in heaven and on earth and under the earth, and every tongue confess that Jesus Christ is Lord, to the glory of God the Father." Paul referred to an Old Testament prophecy in which the verb is much stronger. In Isaiah 45:23, the Lord said, "To me every knee shall bow, every tongue shall swear."

Ultimately, when God calls an end to the kingdoms of this world, every person ever to live will acknowledge that Jesus is Lord of the universe. Even those who to their dying moment denied him will on that day bow to him, acknowledging the supremacy of his power.

But the joy experienced by some will not be shared by all. Thousands, even millions, will be bowing in reverent adoration at the feet of their Savior. Other thousands, even millions, will be bowed low as they are crushed in judgment.

As Revelation 11:15 says of that day, "The kingdom of the world has become the kingdom of our Lord and of his Christ, and he shall reign for ever and ever." We hear those words at Christmas when choral groups heartily sing "The Hallelujah Chorus" from Handel's *Messiah*. But we could very well sing those scriptural words every day of our lives to remind us of the power of our Lord who is one day going to make citizens of his kingdom into beings like himself—new.

All Things New

Even more, he's going to make the world new. Listen to a passage that appears near the end of John's Revelation: "Then I saw a new heaven and a new earth; for the first heaven and the first earth had passed away, and the sea was no more. And I saw the holy city, new Jerusalem, coming down out of heaven from God, prepared as a bride adorned for her husband; and I heard a great voice from the throne saying, 'Behold, the dwelling of God is with men. He will dwell with them, and they shall be his people, and God himself will be with them; he will wipe away every tear from their eyes, and death shall be no more, neither shall there be mourning nor crying nor pain any more, for the former things have passed away.'

"And he who sat upon the throne said, 'Behold, I make all things new'" (21:1–5).

It gives me goose bumps to know that this is what you and I have to look forward to. Why am I so confident that God has prepared such a future kingdom? Verse five continues, "Also he said, 'Write this, for these words are trustworthy and true.'"

Who's that telling the apostle John that these words are trustworthy and true? The One who sits upon the throne: "the Alpha and the Omega, the beginning and the end" (Rev. 21:6); the One who ends his Word to us with an invitation: "Come" (Rev. 22:17). Come into the palace and feast with the king.

"To our God and Father be glory for ever and ever. Amen" (Phil. 4:20).

Jesus Lives!

Jesus lives! thy terrors now
  Can no longer, death, appall us;
Jesus lives! by this we know
  Thou, O grave, canst not enthrall us. Alleluia!

Jesus lives! henceforth is death
  But the gate of life immortal;
This shall calm our trembling breath,
  When we pass its gloomy portal. Alleluia!

Jesus lives! for us he died;
    Then, alone to Jesus living,
Pure in heart may we abide,
    Glory to our Saviour giving. Alleluia!

Jesus lives! our hearts know well
    Naught from us his love shall sever;
Life, nor death, nor powers of hell
    Tear us from his keeping ever. Alleluia!

Jesus lives! to him the throne
    Over all the world is given:
May we go where he has gone,
    Rest and reign with him in heaven. Alleluia!

—C. F. Gellert